PULMONARY FUNCTION TESTING:

A Practical Approach

JACK WANGER, R.R.T., R.C.P.T., M.B.A.

Pulmonary Physiology Unit

National Jewish Center for Immunology

   and Respiratory Medicine

Denver, Colorado

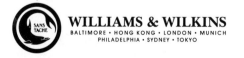

WILLIAMS & WILKINS
BALTIMORE · HONG KONG · LONDON · MUNICH
PHILADELPHIA · SYDNEY · TOKYO

Editor: John P. Butler
Managing Editor: Linda Napora
Copy Editor: Melissa Andrews
Designer: Dan Pfisterer
Illustration Planner: Lorraine Wrzosek
Production Coordinator: Anne Stewart Seitz
Cover Designer: Karen Klinedinst

Copyright © 1992
Williams & Wilkins
428 East Preston Street
Baltimore, Maryland 21202, USA

Accurate indications, adverse reactions, and dosage schedules for drugs are provided in this
book, but it is possible that they may change. The reader is urged to review the package
information data of the manufacturers of the medications mentioned.

Printed in the United States of America

First Edition 1992
Library of Congress Cataloging in Publication Data

Wanger, Jack.
Pulmonary function testing: a practical approach/ Jack Wanger.
   p. cm.
   Includes index.
ISBN 0-683-08607-3
    1. Pulmonary function tests.   I. Title.
   [DNLM: 1. Respiratory Function Tests.   WB 284 W246p]
RC734.P84W36   1992
616.2'40754--dc20
DNLM/DLC
for Library of Congress

91 92 93 94
1 2 3 4 5 6 7 8 9 10

Foreword

"That is a good book which is opened with expectation and closed with profit"

Amos Alcott 1799-1888
American Philosopher and Teacher

Any perusal of a medical bookstore or a bookseller's stall at a medical meeting results in my being overwhelmed by books on the theory and principles of every aspect of lung disease. However, few books take a practical "do-it-yourself" approach—this is one of those books.

I believe that you will find within these pages a wealth of practical information. What you will not find is a lot of hard-to-understand theory and esoterica of little value. I find that too often the students of pulmonary function are confused by symbols (lingo), complex physiological principles and, worst of all—deadly equations! While symbols and equations are found within these pages, they are only the essentials. Most importantly, you will find applicable experiences of and insight into the important concepts presented by someone who has spent years teaching students like yourself.

Note that this book has only five chapters. The first three—spirometry, lung volumes, and diffusing capacity—form what Jack and I term "the ABC's of PFT's." These chapters contain most of what you will need to know about pulmonary function testing and may take you as far as you will need to go. The last two chapters on exercise and bronchial provocation are for those of you who would like to expand your knowledge and the repertoire of your laboratory.

Spirometry should be as commonplace as a blood pressure measurement. To overcome the difficulties encountered in performing this important test, you will find here all the information needed to do it right, information which originates from our teaching experiences in a NIOSH course. Lung volumes are a personal favorite, and we need to credit Reuben Cherniack for engendering in both of us a true appreciation for their measurement. Diffusing capacity is a favorite of Jack's, and I am sure you will see his special insight into its measurement. Exercise testing, especially maximal stress testing, is quite intimidating. Yet, Jack's treatment of this study is clear and utilitarian. Pay special attention to the cases, since I find that students better appreciate exercise testing demonstrated by practical examples. The last chapter, on bronchial provocation, is about our most frequently requested topic and is a "new" addition to many laboratories.

You have before you a practical book and guide to pulmonary function testing. This book represents what it says it does—a practical approach. I know of no more practical person than Jack, and I congratulate him on a wonderful achievement. So, take a big, deep breath and turn the page.

Charlie Irvin, Ph.D.
Denver, Colorado
July 25, 1991

Preface

The field of pulmonary function testing has undergone many changes over the past 20 years. Methods of assessment are undergoing continuous modification and refinement, leading to the development of new techniques and new guidelines on standardization.

Many of the old "workhorses" like the Scholander and Van Slyke analyzers have been swept aside by the constant stream of new and usually improved instruments. The advent of computers has improved quality and increased output.

Although cardiopulmonary technologists have been the mainstays of the pulmonary function laboratory, today, because of the increased awareness of lung disease from smoking and environmental and occupational exposures, we find respiratory therapists, nurses, and industrial hygienists measuring pulmonary function. Often, they have had only minimal classroom instruction; they may have learned their skills from others on the job. They may have sought but not found an appropriate practical "how-to" manual, finding instead that many of the books miss the mark and are intended for the physician or technical director.

This book is intended to be both a practical textbook for students and a reference for those who are performing the tests. I have deliberately excluded various pulmonary function tests (e.g., control of breathing and gas distribution) because I wanted to focus on the most commonly used tests. Additionally, arterial blood gas sampling and analysis are extensively and well covered in other publications.

Each chapter is a self-contained unit that describes and discusses the methods of assessment that are most commonly used today. Each method or group of methods has a brief historical perspective as well as any pertinent background material. The relevant physiology is concisely discussed in practical terms. The instrumentation, techniques, and calculations used are included, as are special considerations such as quality control controversies and basic elements of interpretation. Additionally I have tried to incorporate my experiences in the form of practical hints. The questions at the end of each chapter can be used in the classroom or for self-assessment.

Acknowledgments

In writing this book, I have called on numerous people for advice, help, and support. Their generosity was instrumental in the development of this work.

I first want to express my special and sincere thanks to Pat Brougher for her valuable input, guidance, and encouragement. I am also grateful to Lee Newman, M.D., for his initial encouragement and advice and Karen Rothberg for expert input and critique on the manuscript.

The special illustrations in this book are the result of the outstanding artistic talents and computer capabilities of Leigh Landskroner. I am particularly grateful to her.

My special thanks to Reuben Cherniack, M.D. for his insight and guidance. He has shared his knowledge and continually challenged me to excel.

I also want to express my special thanks to Charles Irvin, Ph.D., who wrote the Foreword of this book. He has been a special friend and colleague over the years and has continually given me encouragement and guidance.

Finally, I want to thank my wife, Betsy, and my daughters, Jessica and Ashley, for their understanding, patience, and tolerance during the preparation of this manuscript.

JACK WANGER

Contents

Pulmonary Terms Symbols, and Definitions

The following terms, symbols, and definitions are taken from the American College of Chest Physicians-American Thoracic Society Joint Committee Statement (Chest 1975;67:583–593).

GASES

V	Gas volume. The particular gas as well as its pressure, water vapor conditions, and other special conditions must be specified in text or indicated by appropriate qualifying symbols.
F	Fractional concentration of gas.
PB	Barometric pressure.
STPD	Standard conditions: Temperature 0°C pressure 760 mm Hg and dry (0 water vapor).
BTPS	Body conditions: Body temperature, ambient pressure, and saturated with water vapor at these conditions.
ATPD	Ambient temperature and pressure, dry.
ATPS	Ambient temperature and pressure, saturated with water vapor at these conditions.
f	Respiratory frequency (breaths per minutes).

t Time.

FORCED SPIROMETRY

FVC Forced vital capacity; vital capacity performed with a maximally forced expiratory effort. This is sometimes referred to as FEVC.

FIVC Forced inspiratory vital capacity; the maximal volume of air inspired with a maximally forced effort from a position of maximal expiration.

FEV₁ Forced expiratory volume in 1 second. The volume of air exhaled in the first second of the FVC. The general symbol is FEVt, where t is the specific time during the performance of the forced vital capacity. Although uncommon, other times besides 1 second are used, for example FEV₂ and FEV₃.

FEV₁/FVC% Forced expiratory volume in 1 second to FVC ratio, as a percent. The general symbol (FEVt/FVC) can be applied for other times (e.g., FEV₃/FVC%).

FEFx Forced expiratory flow, related to some portion of the FVC curve. Modifiers refer to the amount of FVC already exhaled when the measurement is made. For example:
> FEF75%: Instantaneous forced expiratory flow after 75% of the FVC has been exhaled.
> FEF25%: Instantaneous forced expiratory flow after 25% of the FVC has been exhaled.

FEFmax The maximal forced expiratory flow achieved during an FVC. The symbol PEFR is sometimes used to represent this measurement.

PEF The highest forced expiratory flow measured with a peak flow meter.

VmaxX Forced expiratory flow, related to the total lung capacity or the actual volume of the lung at which the measurement is made. *Modifiers refer to amount of lung volume remaining when the* *measurement is made* (e.g., Vmax75% = instantaneous forced expiratory flow when the lung is at 75% of its TLC).

FEF25-75%   Mean forced expiratory flow during the middle half of the FVC.

MVV   Maximal voluntary ventilation. The volume of air expired in a specified period during repetitive maximal respiratory effort at an unrestricted frequency.

FET25-75%   The time required to deliver the FEF25-75%.

FIFx   Forced inspiratory flow. As in the case of the FEF, the appropriate modifiers must be used to designate the volume at which flow is being measured. Unless otherwise specified, the volume qualifiers indicate the volume inspired from RV at the point of the measurement. For example:
  FIF50%: Instantaneous inspiratory flow after 50% of the vital capacity has been inspired from residual volume.

LUNG VOLUMES

RV   Residual volume; that volume of air remaining in the lungs after maximal exhalation, or TLC − VC. The method of measurement should be indicated in the text or, when necessary, by appropriate qualifying symbols.

ERV   Expiratory reserve volume; the maximal volume of air that can be exhaled from the resting end-tidal position.

TV   Tidal volume; that volume of air inhaled or exhaled with each breath during quiet breathing. The symbol TV is used only to indicate a subdivision of lung volume. When tidal volume is used in gas exchange formulations, the symbol V_T should be used.

IRV   Inspiratory reserve volume; the maximal volume of air inhaled from the end-inspiratory level.

IC   Inspiratory capacity; the maximum volume of air that can be inhaled from tidal volume end-expiratory level, or the sum of IRV and TV.

IVC   Inspiratory vital capacity; the maximum volume of air inhaled from the point of maximum expiration.

VC   Vital capacity; the maximum volume of air exhaled from the point of maximum inspiration.

FRC   Functional residual capacity; the volume of air in the lungs at tidal volume end-expiratory level, or the sum of RV and ERV. The method of measurement should be indicated as with RV.

TLC   Total lung capacity; the sum of all volume compartments or the volume of air in the lungs after maximal inspiration. The method of measurement should be indicated.

RV/TLC%   Residual volume to total lung capacity ratio, expressed as a percent.

VA   Alveolar gas volume.

VTG   Thoracic gas volume.

DIFFUSING CAPACITY

Dco   Diffusing capacity of the lung expressed as volume (STPD) of carbon monoxide uptake per unit alveolar-capillary pressure difference. A modifier can be used to designate the technique: e.g., Dco_{sb} is single breath carbon monoxide diffusing capacity. It is also described as **D** and carbon monoxide is assumed to be the test gas. Additionally, the term **DLco** is often used to represent this measurement.

Dm   Diffusing capacity of the alveolar-capillary membrane (STPD).

Θx — Reaction rate coefficient for red cells; the volume STPD of gas (x) that will combine per minute with 1 unit volume of blood per unit gas tension. If the specific gas is not stated, Θ is assumed to refer to CO and is a function of existing O_2 tension.

Qc — Capillary blood volume (usually expressed as Vc in the literature, a symbol inconsistent with those recommended for blood volumes). When determined from the following equation, Qc represents the effective pulmonary capillary blood volume, i.e., capillary blood volume in intimate association with alveolar gas.

Dco/VA — Diffusion of carbon monoxide per unit of alveolar volume with Dco expressed in STPD and VA expressed as liters BTPS.

Dk — Diffusion coefficient or permeability constant as described by Krogh and equals $D(PB-PH_2O)/VA$.

VENTILATION

$\dot{V}E$ — Expired volume per minute (BTPS).

$\dot{V}I$ — Inspired volume per minute (BTPS).

$\dot{V}CO_2$ — Carbon dioxide production per minute (STPD).

$\dot{V}O_2$ — Oxygen consumption per minute (STPD).

$\dot{V}A$ — Alveolar ventilation per minute (BTPS).

$\dot{V}D$ — Ventilation per minute of the physiologic dead space (wasted ventilation, BTPS), defined by the following equation:
$\dot{V}D = \dot{V}E\,(PaCO_2 - PECO_2)\,/\,(PaCO_2 - PICO_2)$.

VD — The physiologic dead space volume defined as $\dot{V}D/f$.

$\dot{V}D_{an}$ — Ventilation per minute of the anatomic dead space, that portion of the conducting airway in which no significant gas exchange occurs (BTPS). VDan is the volume of the anatomic dead space (BTPS).

$\dot{V}$DA

Ventilation of the alveolar dead space (BTPS), defined by the following equation: $\dot{V}DA = \dot{V}D -$ VDan.

$\dot{V}$Aeff

Effective alveolar ventilation defined as $\dot{V}Aeff = \dot{V}E - \dot{V}D$.

$\dot{V}$Drb

Rebreathing ventilation. Ventilation per minute of the rebreathing volume of any external respiratory apparatus (ATPS); or VDrb, the rebreathing volume of an external respiratory device (ATPS).

MECHANICS OF BREATHING

Pressure terms

P

A general symbol for pressure.

Paw

Pressure in the airway, level to be specified.

Pawo

Pressure at the airway opening.

Ppl

Intrapleural pressure.

PA

Alveolar pressure.

PL

Transpulmonary pressure.

Pes

Esophageal pressure used to estimate Ppl.

Flow-pressure relationship terms

R

A general symbol for resistance, pressure per unit flow.

Raw

Airway resistance.

R_L

Total pulmonary resistance, measured by relating flow-dependent transpulmonary pressure to airflow at the mouth.

Rus

Resistance of the airways on the alveolar side (upstream) of the point in the airways where intraluminal pressure equals Ppl, measured under conditions of maximum expiratory flow.

Rds   Resistance of the airways on the oral side (downstream) of the point in the airways where intraluminal pressure equals Ppl.

Gaw   Airway conductance, the reciprocal of Raw.

Gaw/VL   Specific conductance, expressed per liter of lung volume at which G is measured; sometimes referred to as **SGaw**.

Pressure-volume relationship terms

C   A general symbol for compliance, volume change per unit of applied pressure change.

Cdyn   Dynamic compliance, compliance measured at point of zero gas flow at the mouth during active breathing.

Cst   Static compliance, compliance determined from measurements made during conditions of prolonged interruption of air flow.

C/VL   Specific compliance

E   Elastance, pressure per unit of volume change, the reciprocal of compliance.

Pst   Static transpulmonary pressure at a specified lung volume; e.g., PstTLC is static recoil pressure measured at TLC.

PstTLC/TLC   Coefficient of lung retraction expressed per liter of TLC.

W   A general symbol for mechanical work of breathing, which requires use of appropriate qualifying symbols and description of specific conditions.

1

Forced Spirometry

Spirometry is regarded as an essential component in the medical evaluation of patients complaining of shortness of breath. It is also widely used in
patients with allergy problems and in occupational medicine. Although the
utility of spirometry is widely recognized, some obstacles have slowed its
growth: (*a*) inadequate training of personnel, (*b*) technical shortcomings of
certain spirometers, (*c*) lack of standardization of methods, and (*d*) lack of
interpretative skills by physicians.

The American Thoracic Society (ATS) addressed some of these problems in a statement in 1979.[1] These guidelines were the result of recommendations made at a workshop in Snowbird, Utah, in 1977 and became
known as the "Snowbird" recommendations. In 1987, a revised and updated statement was published.[2] This newer version addressed several issues not discussed in the 1979 statement and expanded discussion on such
issues as maneuver performance, measurement reproducibility, and
acceptability.

The purpose of this chapter is to acquaint the student and the practitioner with spirometry and to discuss relevant physiology, instrumentation, techniques of performance and calculations, and basic elements of
interpretation. Because spirometry is frequently assessed before and after bronchodilator, this chapter will also discuss the administration of
bronchodilators.

PHYSIOLOGY

Although the lung is sometimes regarded simply as sort of a bellows system that moves air in and out of the body, it is a complex organ involved in many physiologic processes, including gas transfer between environment and blood and defense against harmful agents (e.g., pollutants), and in biochemical processes that produce substances important in the body.

The lower airways, as shown in Figure 1.1, begin with the trachea and divide into a right and left main stem bronchus. These main stem bronchi (referred to as the first generation of airways) divide into small branches, which become narrower and more numerous as they go deeper into the lung, ending 16 generations later in the primary lobule. Each lobule contains approximately 2200 alveoli.

Inspiration is caused by the contraction of the respiratory muscles. The major respiratory muscle is the diaphragm, and when it contracts, it pushes down toward the abdomen. The other muscles including the external intercostals, scalenes, and sternocleidomastoids increase the lateral and anteroposterior diameter of the thorax.

During quiet breathing, expiration is passive—occurring with relaxation of the respiratory muscles and the return of the lungs and thorax to resting volume. However, during fast, hard breathing, expiration becomes active and the abdominal muscles contract, causing the diaphragm to be pushed upward. Additionally, during fast, hard breathing, the internal intercostal muscles pull the ribs down and inward, decreasing the diameter of the thorax.

During spirometry, the forced expiratory maneuver consists of a maximal inspiration and then a rapid, forceful, and complete expiration. A number of physiologic factors influence the gas flow during this maneuver, but they can be broadly divided into two groups: (*a*) mechanical properties of the lungs and (*b*) resistive elements.

The mechanical properties of the lung refer to the compliance and elastic recoil of the lung. Compliance describes stiffness and is the change in volume of air in the lung divided by the pressure change. Figure 1.2 shows examples of three different pressure volume relationships during a maximum inhalation from functional residual capacity (FRC).

In Figure 1.2*A*, the volume change of 0.5 liter above FRC has a corresponding pressure change of 3 cm H_2O. This means that an additional 3 cm H_2O pressure was required to produce the 0.5-liter volume change. It took approximately 30 cm H_2O of additional pressure to reach maximum inhalation. The compliance of the lung is calculated by dividing the volume

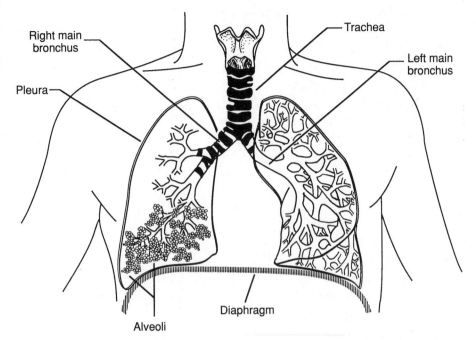

Figure 1.1. Larynx, trachea, main stem bronchi, and branches developing to the alveoli.

change by the transpulmonary pressure change, which in this example equals 0.17 liter/cm H_2O. This would be an example of normal compliance.

In Figure 1.2*B*, the volume change of 0.5 liter above FRC has a corresponding pressure change of 9 cm H_2O, equaling a compliance of 0.06 liter/cm H_2O. This would be an example of stiff lungs as found in various forms of pulmonary fibrosis.

In Figure 1.2*C*, the volume change of 0.5 liter above FRC has a corresponding pressure change of 1.5 cm H_2O, equaling a compliance of 0.33 liter/cm H_2O. This would be an example of overly compliant lungs as found in patients with emphysema.

Elastic recoil refers to the tendency of the lungs to return to their resting or relaxed state. The more the lung tissue is stretched, the stronger will be the elastic recoil and the higher the maximal flow in the airways. Thus the elastic recoil pressure and maximal flow are greatest when the lungs are fully inflated and the least when the lungs are nearly emptied. Elastic recoil will also vary with disease. In patients with emphysema, there is lower elastic recoil because of the loss of tissue. In patients with pulmonary fibrosis (stiff lungs), the elastic recoil is increased.

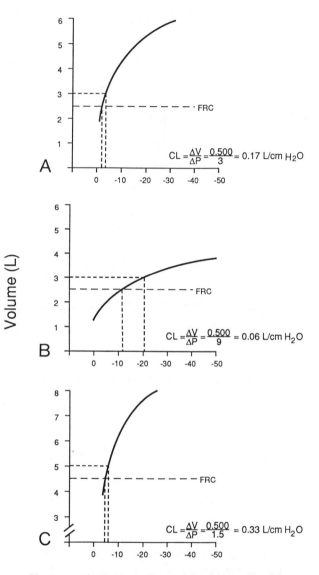

$$CL = \frac{\Delta V}{\Delta P} = \frac{0.500}{3} = 0.17 \text{ L/cm H}_2\text{O}$$

$$CL = \frac{\Delta V}{\Delta P} = \frac{0.500}{9} = 0.06 \text{ L/cm H}_2\text{O}$$

$$CL = \frac{\Delta V}{\Delta P} = \frac{0.500}{1.5} = 0.33 \text{ L/cm H}_2\text{O}$$

Transpulmonary Pressure (cm H$_2$O)

Figure 1.2. Three pressure volume curves illustrating the relationship between transpulmonary pressure and volume. **A** shows a pressure volume curve where the change in volume divided by the change in pressure between FRC and 0.5 liter above FRC is in the normal range of 0.12 to 0.25 L/cm H$_2$O. **B** shows a pressure volume curve where the change in volume divided by the change in pressure between FRC and 0.5 liter above FRC is lower than the normal range as might be seen in individuals with stiff lungs (e.g., pulmonary fibrosis). **C** shows a pressure volume curve where the change in volume divided by the change in pressure between FRC and 0.5 liter above FRC is higher than the normal range as might be seen in individuals with overly compliant lungs (e.g., emphysema).

The second major factor that influences gas flow is the resistance to airflow. The caliber of the conducting airways plays the major role. The smaller the diameter of the conducting airway, the more the resistance. There are two main factors affecting the caliber of the airway. The first is the lung volume. The airways are wider and longer at full inspiration than toward the end of expiration, which is why patients who have airflow limitation often breathe at higher lung volumes. The second factor affecting the caliber of the airway is contraction of the bronchial smooth muscles. As they are stimulated via receptors, these muscles contract, reducing the airway caliber.

Airway collapsibility also affects the caliber of the airway and is best explained by the pressure-flow relationship and the single equal-pressure-point model (Fig. 1.3). When there is no flow in the airways, the alveolar pressure and the airway pressure are equal and approximately atmospheric. During an inspiration, alveolar and pleural pressures become subatmospheric and air rushes into the lungs. During expiration, alveolar and pleural pressures become positive and exceed atmospheric pressure. During a forced expiration this pressure change is amplified as shown in Figure 1.3. The airways are forced to narrow at the point when the pressure in the thorax becomes greater than the airway pressure. The point where these two pressures (thorax and airway) are exactly equal is called the equal pressure point (EPP). The airways on the alveolar side of the EPP are referred to as the "upstream airways," and those on the mouth side of the EPP are called the "downstream airways."

The maximal flow that can be achieved is explained mathematically by the following formula:

$$\text{Maximal flow} = \frac{\text{Pressure change}}{\text{Resistance}}$$

Thus increases in elastic recoil pressure without increases in resistance result in increases in maximal flow. Likewise, increases in resistance usually reduce maximal flow.

INSTRUMENTATION

Available spirometers can be classified as either (*a*) **volume displacing** or (*b*) **flow sensing.** Before discussing these two broad groups, the reader should also know at this point that there are two types of

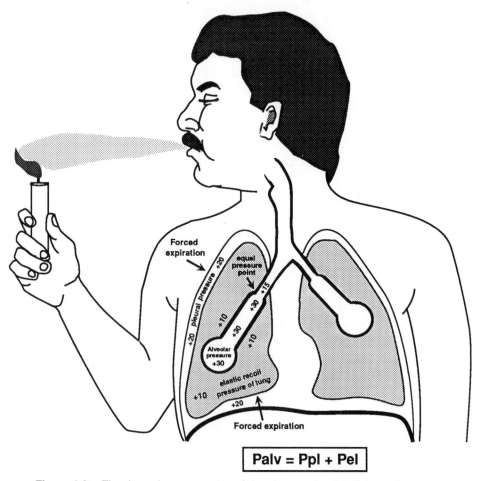

$$\boxed{\text{Palv} = \text{Ppl} + \text{Pel}}$$

Figure 1.3. The dynamic compression of the airways showing the equal pressure point (EPP). During the forced expiration the respiratory muscles compress the thorax. Alveolar pressure (Palv), in this case 30 cm H_2O, is the sum of the pleural pressure (in this case Ppl = 20 cm H_2O) and the elastic recoil pressure (in this case Pel = 10 cm H_2O). The pressure in the airways falls as the mouth is approached. When the pleural pressure equals alveolar pressure the EPP is reached. Downstream from that point (toward the mouth) the airways narrow limiting airflow.

graphic displays that can be displayed from either of these two groups of spirometers: volume-time and flow-volume. Figure 1.4 shows a **volume-time curve** with volume (in liters) on the Y-axis and time (in seconds) on the X-axis. Figure 1.5 shows a **flow-volume curve** with flow (in liters/second) on the Y-axis and volume (in liters) on the X-axis.

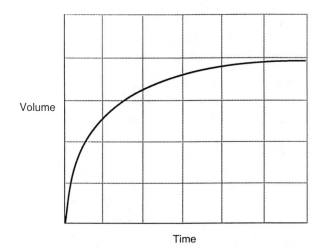

Time

Figure 1.4. The volume-time curve as might be seen during a forced vital capacity maneuver. The advantage of this display is the ability to view small changes in volume as the maneuver ends, thus helping the technician to better detect the end of the test.

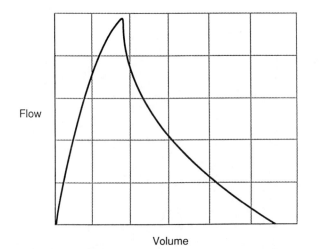

Volume

Figure 1.5. The flow-volume curve as might be seen during a forced vital capacity maneuver. The advantage of this display is the ability to see peak flow (which provides information on patient effort and technique at the start of the test) and better view abnormalities pictorially.

Volume-Displacing Spirometers

WATER-SEAL, BELLOWS, ROLLING-SEAL, DIAPHRAGM

The volume-displacement spirometer has a very long history and was the type John Hutchinson used in his experiments in 1850. The volume-dis-

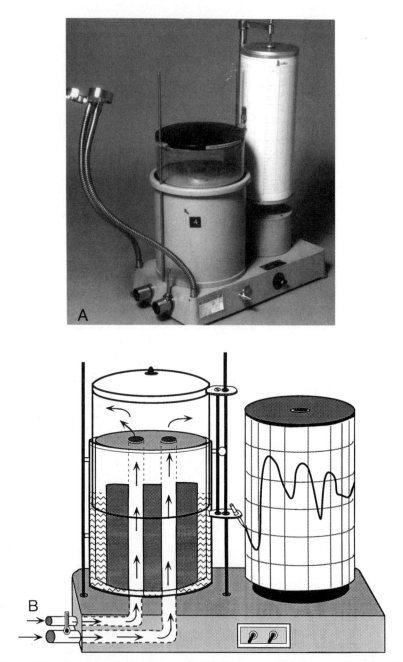

Figure 1.6. **A** shows the water-sealed Stead-Wells spirometer as a unit (photograph by Barry Silverstein) and **B** shows how the air moves into and out of the spirometer bell and keeps from escaping.

placement spirometer collects exhaled air or acts as a reservoir for inhaled air. Figure 1.6*A* and *B* show a Stead-Wells spirometer, which is considered to be the "gold standard." This spirometer consists of three cylinders: an outer hollow cylinder open on the top, a second cylinder approximately ½ inch smaller in diameter and closed on the top except for one or two large holes, and a third cylinder of lightweight plastic with its open bottom placed into the space between the first and second cylinders. The space between the first and second cylinders is also filled with water. The third cylinder (sometimes called the bell) moves up and down in the water when a patient is connected. When the patient exhales into the mouthpiece and the tubing, exhaled air forces the bell upward. The water acts as a seal and keeps this air from escaping—a water seal. A pen connected to the bell writes on paper affixed to a rotating drum (the kymograph).

The bellows type spirometer is another example of the volume-displacement spirometer. Exhaled air is collected in a bellow, much like the one used to "coax" flames from fireplace coals. Bellows spirometers are usually made of plastic, and the material expands as exhaled air enters and contracts as air exits. The vertical bellows, or wedge spirometer, shown in Figures 1.7 and 1.8, is large and bulky and was popular in the 1960s and 1970s. The horizontal bellows shown in Figures 1.9 and 1.10 is smaller and more practical and is in wide use today. Both of these bellows systems can display results electronically with a computer or microprocessor or mechanically with a pen and kymograph.

The dry rolling-seal spirometer is the third type of volume-displacement spirometer (shown in Figs. 1.11 and 1.12). The piston-in-cylinder can be vertical or horizontal. A silicone-based elastic material seals the spirometer contents by rolling with the piston as it moves (thus the name *rolling-seal spirometer*). The volume is measured by a potentiometer that is mechanically connected to the piston rod with a slide wire. Flow data are obtained by electronic differentiation of the volume signal. Like the bellows spirometer, the rolling-seal spirometer can also display results electronically or mechanically with a pen.

The fourth type of volume-displacement spirometer, one that incorporates a diaphragm, is shown in Figure 1.13. Such spirometers are small, lightweight, and simple to use and can be purchased with or without a microprocessor. As shown in Figure 1.13, the patient breathing tube connects to the bottom of the unit. A rubber diaphragm fits snugly into the lower housing. As the patient's exhaled air enters the lower housing, it pushes the bottom side of the diaphragm upward. As the diaphragm moves upward, it pushes a pusher plate upward, and volume is then measured.

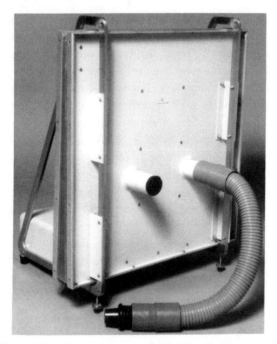

Figure 1.7.   The wedge spirometer—a vertical bellows spirometer. (Photograph by Barry Silverstein.)

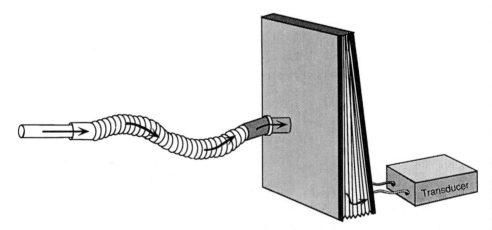

Figure 1.8.   The vertical bellows type spirometer illustrating how the bellowslike action collects exhaled air and senses movement.

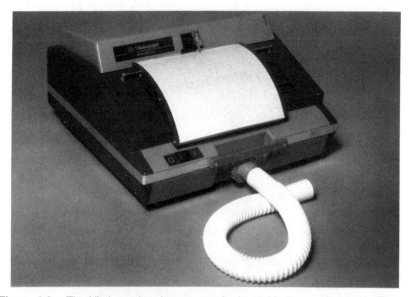

Figure 1.9. The Vitalograph spirometer—a horizontal bellows spirometer. (Photograph by Barry Silverstein.)

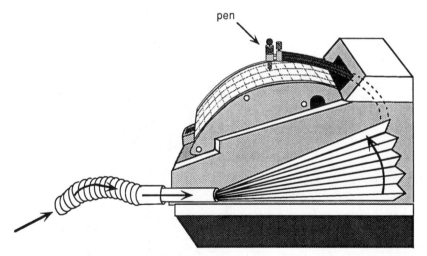

Figure 1.10. The horizontal bellows type spirometer illustrating how the bellows collects expired air and records the volume.

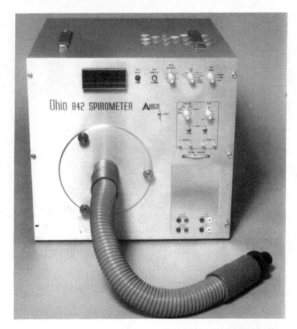

Figure 1.11.   The Ohio rolling-seal spirometer. (Photograph by Barry Silverstein.)

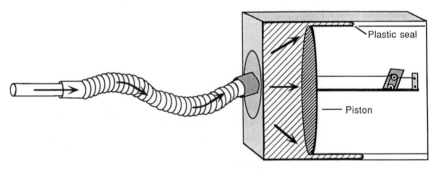

Figure 1.12.   The rolling-seal spirometer illustrating how the piston-cylinder mechanism collects and seals exhaled air.

The exhaled air escapes back out of the patient breathing tube when the patient's mouth is removed. A volume-time tracing can be obtained, and if the instrument is equipped with a microprocessor, this device will calculate several parameters.

The volume-displacing spirometers are generally designed to measure exhaled volumes and, prior to commencement of the test, contain no air. However, the water-seal and vertical bellow spirometers do allow the user to add air by moving the resting position. This allows the

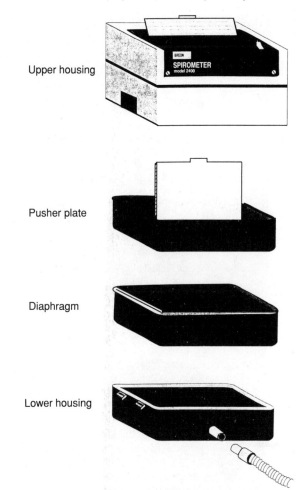

Figure 1.13. The diaphragm-type spirometer, which collects exhaled air beneath a diaphragm, which pushes upward on a pusher-plate and writing mechanism.

patient both to inhale deeply from the reservoir and to exhale completely.

The major pitfall with volume-displacing spirometers is that they can develop leaks. If they leak, volume cannot be collected accurately. Therefore, one of the most important quality control activities is to "leak test" these devices. This can be done at the time of calibration on some types, but on others it may take a bit more ingenuity.

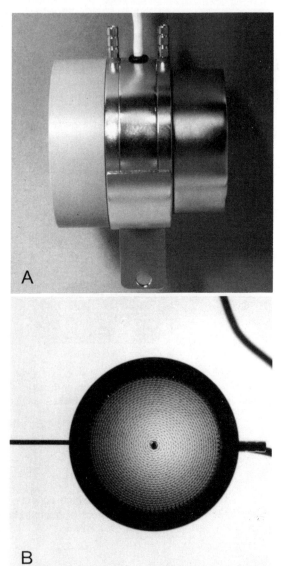

Figure 1.14. The Fleisch pneumotach (a differential pressure flow-sensing device) from the side, **A**, and from the front, **B**, showing the honey-combed resistive element. (Photographs by Barry Silverstein.)

Summary of characteristics of volume-displacing spirometers

Desirable
Directly measures volume
Low cost
Ease of operation
Water-seal spirometer is considered to be the "gold standard"

Possibly Undesirable
Some are very large and bulky
Less portable
Water in water-seal devices needs changing
Leaks
Without microprocessor or computer, manual calculations are necessary

---

Flow-Sensing Spirometers

The shortcomings of volume-displacing spirometers (e.g., large, bulky, frequency response issues) led to the development of the flow-sensing devices.

Flow-sensing spirometers directly measure flow. Volume is calculated by multiplying flow by time, which is known as "integration." This process requires a computer or microprocessor. The four major types of airflow measuring devices are (*a*) differential pressure device, (*b*) thermistor or hot-wire anemometer, (*c*) turbine device, and (*d*) vortex device.

Examples of the **differential pressure** device or **pneumotachygraph** or **pneumotach** are shown in Figures 1.14 and 1.15. The device consists of a tube with fixed resistance. The fixed resistance, which is very small and not sensed by the patient, can be a bundle of capillary tubes running parallel to the flow (Fleisch type) or a fine mesh screen or set of screens. As air flows through the tube in either direction, it meets the fixed resistance. The pressure on the side from which flow originates becomes greater than the pressure on the other side. The greater the flow the greater the pressure difference. The pressure difference is measured with a pressure transducer, and the signal is sent electronically to amplifiers and then to a computer or microprocessor.

The relationship among flow, pressure, and resistance can be explained mathematically with the following formula:

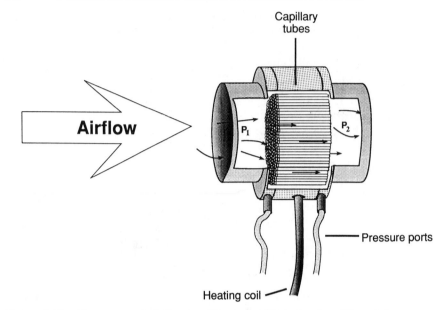

Figure 1.15. The pneumotach flow-sensing device illustrating the differential pressure principle. As airflow enters the pneumotach it meets the resistive element. The pressure on the airflow side of the element (P_1) is greater than the pressure on the other side of the resistive element (P_2). The two pressures are transmitted via the pressure ports to a transducer, which is connected to electronic amplifiers and computers or recorders. The heating coil heats the resistive element to reduce moisture buildup, and, if heated to 37°C, it measures airflow at body temperature.

$$\text{Flow} = \frac{\text{Pressure}}{\text{Resistance}}$$

The accuracy of a pneumotachygraph depends on the maintenance of a fixed resistance across the capillary tubes or screens. One can see from the above formula that with a fixed resistance, pressure is directly proportional to flow. However if the resistance increases (e.g., secretions or exhaled water vapor collects on the screens or in the capillary tubes), this relationship changes and flow can be incorrectly measured. Some pneumotachygraphs incorporate a heater (37°C) to prevent condensation; others use a longer patient tube between the mouth and the pneumotach to trap the condensed moisture and secretions so that resistance across the screen or capillary tubes remains unchanged.

The **thermistor** or **hot-wire anemometer** consists of a fine piece of wire in the center of a tube as shown in Figure 1.16. As air moves through the

Heated wire

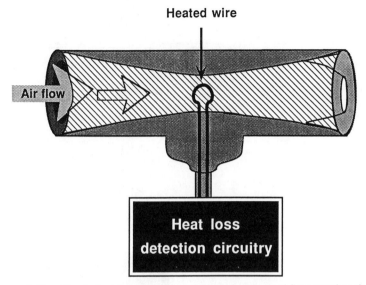

Air flow

**Heat loss
detection circuitry**

Figure 1.16. The hot-wire anemometer (thermistor) type of flow-sensing device.

tube, it cools the heated wire. Electrical energy reheats the wire and maintains it at a specific temperature. The current, which raises with the airflow, is measured, electronically linearized, and read as flow through the device.

There are some problems with hot-wire devices. Turbulent flow cannot be measured accurately, and laminar flow must be ensured by providing a long tube between the patient and the hot-wire housing. Also, the heated wire is fragile and responds to movement when the device is handheld.

A **turbine** device is shown in Figure 1.17. The speed of the turbine (i.e., rotating wheel) increases as airflow increases. An electronic circuit counts the revolutions and calculates flow. The accuracy of the device is not affected by turbulent flow, water vapor, or gas composition, but the inertia of the turbine introduces inaccuracies with changing airflows. Newer designs have tried to improve on this problem by decreasing the weight of the rotating vanes.

The **vortex** device (shown in Fig. 1.18) is based on the principle that air flowing through a tube becomes turbulent when it meets obstructions. Struts or obstructing protrusions fixed in the breathing tube cause swirling or turbulence in gas flowing through the tube. Each individual swirl is called a "vortex." Each vortex is counted by an ultrasonic beam, and a specific volume is applied. Vortex devices have a major weakness in that they are not sensitive enough to always measure low flow rates.

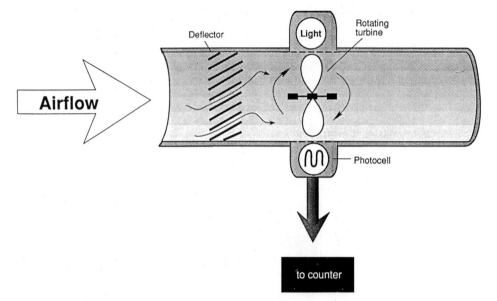

Figure 1.17. The turbine or rotating type of flow-sensing device.

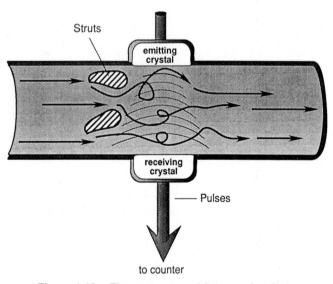

Figure 1.18. The vortex type of flow-sensing device.

Summary of characteristics of flow-sensing spirometers

Desirable
Smaller and usually more portable
Computerized, thus no manual calculations
Computerization also provides quick reference values
Bidirectional devices provide flow volume loop capability

Possibly Undesirable
More knowledge needed to operate computer or microprocessor
Frequent and careful calibration needed
Moisture condensation can cause problems
Gas composition can affect results
May not sense low flows

What Spirometer to Choose for Your Needs?

The ATS first published recommendations for spirometer standards in 1979[1] and updated those recommendations in 1987.[2] Manufacturers are aware of these specification standards and appear to attempt to comply with them. However, the reader should be aware of some of the specific standards before selecting a spirometer for his or her needs.

If the spirometer measures forced vital capacity (FVC), it should be able to measure volumes of at least 7 liters and flow rates (both inspiratory and expiratory) between 0 and 12 liters/second. Although it is rare to find patients with greater than 7 liters vital capacity, they do exist. Also, one rarely sees maximum flow rates greater than 16 liters/second, but many healthy individuals can achieve flows in the 12 to 16 liters/second range. Prolonged exhalation times are seen in obstructed patients and, therefore, the spirometer should be able to accumulate volume for at least 15 seconds. If the spirometer is to be used to measure FEV_1, the operator should be able to determine start of test by the back extrapolation technique, which I will discuss later.

A recent evaluation of spirometers found that 12% of the spirometers did not accurately measure a 3-liter calibration syringe, and 29% of the spirometers performed "unacceptably" when an FVC simulator introduced 24 different waveforms. Additionally, this evaluation found software errors in 25% of the computerized systems.[3]

Table 1.1: General types of spirometers that can be purchased based on answers to "needs" questions

	Noncomputerized Volume Displacement	Computerized Volume Displacement	Flow Sensing
User knowledge	Low	Higher	Higher
Number of tests/day	<10	1–40	1–40
Amount of pulmonary function data	FVC, FEV$_1$	More than FVC and FEV$_1$	More than FVC and FEV$_1$
Speed of calculations	Slow	Fast	Fast
Cost	Low	High	High
Portability	No	Yes	Yes

The companies that make and design the spirometers in use today are continually developing new devices or modifying and upgrading existing ones. Users usually benefit from this development and upgrading process and from the competition among companies. I will not recommend specific brands or types but will present a method designed to enable the user to decide what is best for a particular application. This method starts with some questions:

1. Who will conduct the tests, and what is their level of knowledge? Do they have experience with computers? Can they calculate values by hand?
2. How many tests per day will be performed?
3. What pulmonary function values are needed? Will FVC and FEV$_1$ be enough, or will other values such as inspiratory flows be needed?
4. How quickly are the results needed—immediately or within an hour or two?
5. How much money is available?
6. Must the system be portable?

If one first answers these questions and then determines which devices under consideration meet the ATS equipment recommendations, a better determination can be made of spirometry needs. Table 1.1 presents my recommendations for spirometer types based on the answers to the above questions.

Once the user has decided on a type of spirometer, there is still a decision to be made on which brand to purchase. The criteria that should be examined in that decision include price, service, ease of cleaning, delivery time, and, in the case of computerized models, the "friendliness" of the software.

The user should request a demonstrator unit to allow evaluation. The evaluation process should consist of at least the following:

1. Check specifications against ATS requirements.
2. Use a known-volume calibration syringe to inject and/or withdraw known volumes at different speeds. This step should not be done in the calibration mode but one in which a patient's interaction is simulated. The results from the instrument will be body temperature and pressure saturated (BTPS), which means that if you use a 3-liter syringe, the reported FVC should be approximately 3.3 liters (BTPS).
3. Test yourself and/or other laboratory staff and simulate "problem" patients. For example, perform a poor start of test and an early termination to observe the instrument's response. Does it warn you about back extrapolation error? Does it start prematurely from moving the tube around? Does it end the trial prematurely?
4. If possible, compare computerized FVC and FEV$_1$ values to hand-calculated values.
5. Ask the salesperson for the names of other users who have purchased the instrument. Call or write them and ask their opinion and experiences.
6. If possible, subject it to a device that produces a set of standard waveforms.[2]

Although purchasing is the most common option, some companies or hospitals provide the user with a leased spirometer, phone modem, and training. The user, in return, pays a per-test fee for a pulmonologist's interpretation and inspection of the results. This is referred to as an **outreach** program and is becoming more popular, especially in areas where a pulmonologist is not available.

Calibration

Spirometers, like other monitoring and diagnostic instruments, can generate erroneous information. **However, if they are calibrated and leak tested (volume-displacing spirometers) every day of use, the likelihood of errors is greatly reduced.**

Every laboratory or office should obtain a **calibration syringe** (shown in Fig. 1.19) with a volume of at least 3 liters that has been checked against a standard. In 1991, the price range of these syringes was $300 to $500.

Volume-displacing spirometers should have the patient testing tube attached during calibration so it too can be included in the leak testing process (Fig. 1.20). Visual inspection alone may not reveal tears resulting from use and cleaning.

The procedure for calibrating and leak testing the volume-displacing spirometer is easy. Inject the entire syringe volume and observe the spirometer or mechanical pen tracing. If the bell falls or the pen line does not

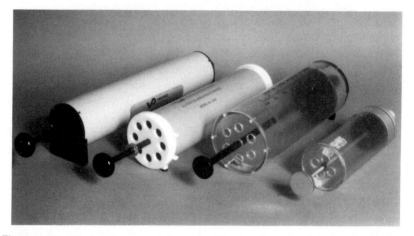

Figure 1.19. Various types and sizes of calibration (known-volume) syringes. (Photograph by Barry Silverstein.)

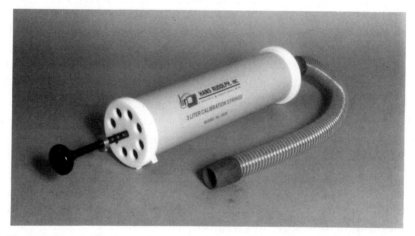

Figure 1.20. Calibration syringe using the patient breathing tube. (Photograph by Barry Silverstein.)

travel in a straight line (Fig. 1.21), a leak is present. Locating and repairing leaks should be done by knowledgeable staff. **If no leak is present, the volume shown on the chart paper or on the computer should equal the syringe volume within ±3%.** For example, if a 3-liter syringe is being used, the acceptable range would be 2.91 to 3.09 liters. Some companies recommend injecting the syringe volume several times at different speeds; the user should follow these recommendations as stated in the spirometer user manual.

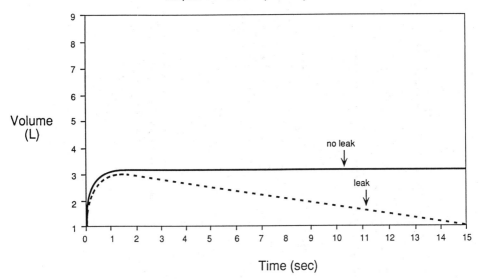

Figure 1.21. A volume-time trace illustrating a proper calibration and leak test (*solid line*) of a volume-displacement spirometer with a 3-liter calibration syringe, and an unacceptable calibration and leak test (*dashed line*).

Flow-sensing spirometers usually have a calibration selection among the "menu" options. Again, some companies recommend several injections at different speeds, and these recommendations should be followed. However, at least one injection of the known volume calibration syringe should be done, and the measured value must be within the ±3%. When injecting at different speeds, the ATS suggests emptying the syringe in 0.5 to 1 second, 1 to 1.5 seconds, and 5 to 5.5 seconds.

If the spirometer is unable to measure the calibration syringe volume within ±3%, the spirometer should not be used until it is serviced or repaired.

A calibration log or notebook should be established for each spirometer. The date and time, expected or known volume, measured volume, and technician initials should be entered. Some computerized models allow the user to print a page with all this information. This log is useful in verifying that the device was calibrated and for noting trends that may indicate equipment problems.

Quality Control

Along with calibration each day there are a couple of other suggestions that will help ensure quality.

1. **Laboratory Standards:** Choose two or three laboratory workers who are healthy nonsmokers to serve as "laboratory standards." Gather spirometry data on each person and record the results in a quality control or calibration notebook. Repeat this procedure four times per year, keeping a mean and coefficient of variation (standard deviation/mean) for several parameters (e.g., FVC and FEV_1). If on a quarterly test or at other times when the spirometer data are suspect, the standard's values deviate from the past values by a coefficient of variation of more than 5%, the spirometer should be serviced and not used until it again reads correctly.

2. **Recorder Time Sweep:** If the spirometer is a volume-displacement device that has a recorder with a time sweep, the speed must be checked against a stopwatch.

3. **Entire Range:** Volume-displacement spirometers should be checked over their entire range using the calibration syringe. Another option is to calibrate this type of spirometer at other starting points besides the zero position and check against the chart paper.

SPIROMETRIC TECHNIQUE

Because spirometry is effort dependent, and its validity is grounded in its reproducibility, successful spirometry requires the application of a consistent **technique** for preparing the patient, explaining and performing the procedure, and inspecting and accepting or rejecting the results.

Patient Preparation

In many hospitals and offices, patient preparation really begins when the patient is scheduled. At that time, the patient is usually instructed on such things as which medications should be withheld (if any), whether he/she should stop smoking for a specific period of time, and possibly others.

When the patient arrives in the laboratory for testing, patient preparation consists of explaining the purpose of the test, determining if there are any contraindications to performing spirometry, obtaining height and weight, positioning the patient, and explaining the actual maneuver.

Whenever a patient visits a physician's office or hospital laboratory for a new procedure, that individual is usually anxious or fearful of what lies ahead. Is it going to hurt? Are they going to "poke" a needle in my arm? Is it going to take a long time? These and other questions are going through the patient's mind, and therefore a brief explanation of the test, how it will be done, and what purpose it has is important. Keep the explanation of spirometry in simple terms and be brief. Do not try to second-guess the ordering physician (e.g., questioning the orders for spirometry or type of bronchodilator) in front of the patient, and do not make statements that make the patient more uncomfortable. One statement that works well is "I am going to have you blow into a machine to see how big your lungs are and how fast the air comes out. It doesn't hurt, but it will require your cooperation and lots of effort."

Spirometry can be significantly influenced by the condition of the patient. Therefore, postponement of testing for an hour or two, for a day, or even for several weeks is not out of the question. Several important criteria that would contraindicate spirometry are (*a*) the patient recently took a bronchodilator and the spirometry is ordered for "before and after bronchodilator"; (*b*) a recent viral infection (within 2 to 3 weeks) or other acute illness, especially when occupational or other screenings are being done for longitudinal studies (comparisons over time); (*c*) a serious illness such as recent myocardial infarction, pulmonary emboli, etc.; and (*d*) cigarettes or a heavy meal within an hour of testing.

Spirometric results are often compared to reference or predicted values. In order to do this correctly, the patient's height (without shoes), age (on day of test), and, sometimes, weight are needed. In patients with spinal deformities and those who cannot stand, the measurement of arm span closely equals standing height.[4]

Getting the patient comfortable and in the proper position is the next important step. Have the patient loosen any tight clothing like neckties, belts, or bras. There is no significant difference in results between the sitting and standing positions, so have the patient do what is most comfortable or convenient. When using the sitting position, which offers the benefit of support in case of loss of balance, be sure the patient's legs are uncrossed and both feet are on the floor.

Explaining the actual maneuver is the last step in the patient preparation process. The patient should be shown the mouthpiece and noseclips (which should always be worn). Explain how the mouthpiece fits into the mouth. In the case of cardboard mouthpieces, be sure to tell the patient not to bite down, as this will obstruct the tubing hole. Lips should be sealed tightly and the tongue should not stick out into the mouthpiece. Dentures that fit poorly may be a nuisance and should be removed if it is thought they interfere.

Show the patient the proper chin and neck position. As shown in Figure 1.22, the chin should be slightly elevated and the neck slightly extended. This position should be maintained throughout the forced expiratory procedure. Don't let the patient bend the chin to the chest. Some

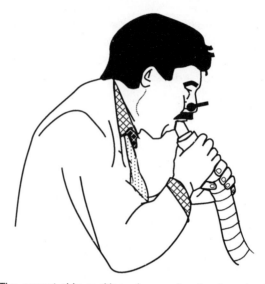

Figure 1.22. The correct chin position when performing forced spirometry. Note that the chin is not bent excessively toward the chest.

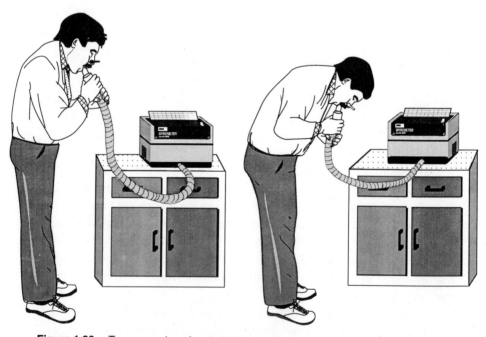

Figure 1.23. Two examples of an individual performing forced spirometry. **A** shows the correct posture, and **B** illustrates too much bending of neck and chin.

bending at the waist is common and acceptable, but discourage bending all the way over (Fig. 1.23).

The specific instructions on the maneuver should be in simple terms. For example, "I want you to take the deepest breath possible, put the mouthpiece in your mouth and seal your lips tightly, and then blast all your air into the tube as hard and as fast as you can in one long complete breath." For spirometers that allow the patient to already be breathing on the mouthpiece, the instructions would be simpler. One analogy that is sometimes helpful to further explain the maneuver is "It's like blowing out the candles on a birthday cake and they all don't go out, so you need to keep blowing in the same breath until they do."

Next, demonstrate the maneuver. Many patients will forget some or all of the instructions they just received, so the demonstration reinforces exactly what they are to do. Show the patient proper chin and neck position, how to get the mouthpiece in at the right time, and how to blast the air out and continue blowing.

When the demonstration is done, remind the patient on a few key points: "Be sure to take as deep a breath as possible, blast out hard, and don't stop blowing until I tell you." If inspiratory flow volume curves are desired, remind the patient to inhale deeply and as fast as possible.

Summary of important points for procedure explanation

1. *Keep the explanation in simple terms and don't be wordy.*
2. *Demonstrate the maneuver.*
3. *Remind the patient of key points.*
4. *Give the patient feedback after the maneuver.*

Performance and Inspection of the Maneuver

The technician should use good active and forceful coaching in having the patient perform the maneuver (Fig. 1.24). The technician needs to raise his/her voice with some urgency, using such phrases as "blow, blow, blow," "keep blowing, keep blowing," and "don't stop blowing." Coaching improves the performance of most effort dependent activities including spirometry. After a maneuver give the patient some feedback on the quality of the test and describe what improvements could be made. Continue to repeat efforts until **three acceptable maneuvers** are obtained. If after eight trials no acceptable curves are obtained, it is reasona-

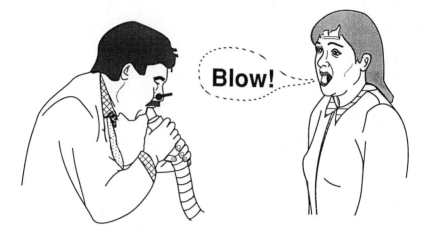

Figure 1.24.   Use good coaching during forced spirometry.

ble to stop and report that the patient could not perform acceptable spirometry.

Acceptability with regard to spirometric maneuvers consists of five characteristics: (*a*) no coughing, (*b*) good start of test, (*c*) no early termination, (*d*) no variable flows, and (*e*) consistency. Let's look at each of these criteria in more detail.

The maneuver should contain **no coughing**, especially during the first second. Many patients, however, commonly cough with each effort toward the end of the test. If this is the case, the technician should note that the patient coughed with each trial and that's all that could be obtained. Figure 1.25 shows some examples of spirograms where the patient coughed.

There must be a **good start of test.** The beginning of the forced expiratory maneuver is extremely important in calculating many parameters. Therefore, the start of the test must be quick and forceful. An unsatisfactory start of test is characterized by excessive hesitation or the extrapolated volume (discussed later in calculations) is greater than 5% of the FVC or 100 ml, whichever is greater. Figure 1.26 shows both a volume-time and flow-volume display of efforts that had a poor start of test. When patients demonstrate this problem, the technician needs to remind the patient about "blasting out" and not hesitating.

Occasionally the technician questions the efforts of a patient because the individual appears not to be blowing as hard or as fast as he/she can, or the peak flow rates are variable between maneuvers. Because submaximal efforts can result in errors and variability in the FEV$_1$, peak expiratory flow

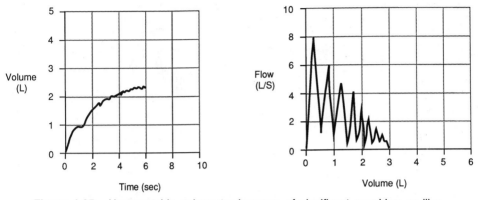

Figure 1.25. Unacceptable spirometry because of significant coughing as illustrated in the volume-time and flow-volume spirograms.

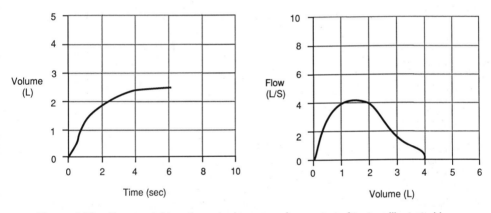

Figure 1.26. Unacceptable spirometry because of poor start of test as illustrated in the volume-time and flow-volume spirograms. Note the rounded shape of the flow-volume graph at the highest point (peak flow).

rate (PEFR), and other measurements, I teach a technique that helps the technician determine whether or not a patient is blowing out as fast as he/she can at the beginning of the test. This technique is to have the patient take a deep breath and cough into the spirometer tube (only a small amount of air needs to be coughed out, not the entire vital capacity). The resulting cough peak expiratory flow rate represents a good approximation of the peak flow that should be obtained when the patient is asked to "blow the air out as fast and as hard as you can." If the difference between the cough PEFR and the forced vital capacity PEFR is more than 1 liter/second, poor patient effort or technique should be suspected.

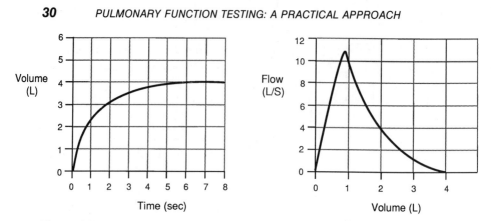

Figure 1.27. Acceptable spirometry. Volume-time spirogram illustrates the expiratory plateau with no change in volume for at least 2 seconds.

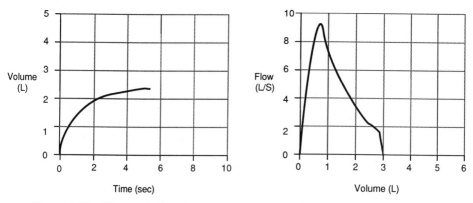

Figure 1.28. Unacceptable spirometry because of no plateau as in the volume-time graph. Note the "cliff" at the end of the flow-volume graph indicating an abrupt end to flow.

No early termination of expiration is another acceptability criterion. There must be a minimum exhalation time of 6 seconds unless there is an obvious plateau (no change in volume for at least 2 seconds) on volume-time displays (Fig. 1.27). On flow-volume displays, the computer or microprocessor should alert the technician as to when the end of the test occurs (usually a "beep"). However, some of these devices "beep" when the flow drops below a certain threshold. Just because it "beeps" does not necessarily mean that the entire vital capacity has been exhaled (Fig. 1.28). In fact, a patient could stop halfway through and the instrument would beep. The technician must pay close attention to the expiratory time and should coach the patient to blow at least 6 seconds up to a maximum of 15 to 20 seconds (some patients can blow longer than 15 to 20 seconds, but the amount of volume collected beyond that point is probably not clinically significant). Not meeting this criterion is frequently the result of poor coaching, so keep urging the patient to "keep blowing, keep blowing, don't stop yet, keep blowing."

The spirogram **should not have variable flow rates.** This means the flow should be consistent and as fast as possible throughout the exhaled vital capacity. Figure 1.29 shows an example of variable flow.

The final acceptability criterion is that of **reproducibility (consistency) of efforts.** Because spirometry is an effort-dependent test, reproducible FVCs and FEV$_1$s occur if the patient is trying as hard as he/she can during each effort. The two largest FVCs and FEV$_1$s should agree within 5% or 100 ml, whichever is greater. Figure 1.30 demonstrates three acceptable spirometric curves where the two largest agree within 5%. Figure 1.31 demonstrates an unacceptable set of spirometry curves, and thus, more efforts need to be obtained.

Occasionally, a patient will have spirometry-induced bronchospasm, meaning that each effort is worse in terms of airflow than the previous one. Most patients with this characteristic eventually will stop getting worse with each trial and will reach a plateau, but he/she may be too short of breath at that point to go on. An interesting problem arises when spirometry worsens with each effort. Which effort should be selected for the final report? The best effort (1) in Figure 1.32 is frequently chosen because it has the best numbers, but if before-and-after bronchodilator studies are being done, the worst effort (4) would be more appropriate.

Inspiratory curves or "loops" have not been addressed by the ATS for acceptability standards. However, two criteria to consider are (*a*) that the inspiratory vital capacity be ≥95% of the expiratory vital capacity and (*b*) that the peak inspiratory flows agree within 1 liter/second.

Summary of acceptability criteria

---

1. No coughing, especially during first second
2. Good start of test
3. No early termination of expiration
4. No variable flows
5. Good reproducibility or consistency of efforts

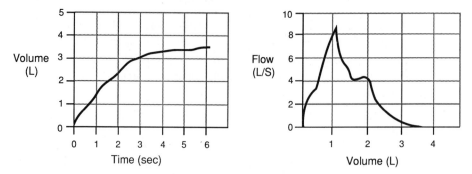

Figure 1.29. Unacceptable spirometry because of variable flow rates. Patients must be coached and instructed to blow as fast and as hard as possible throughout the test.

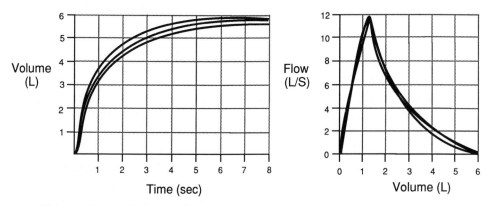

Figure 1.30. Acceptable spirometry as illustrated with volume-time and flow-volume graphs. Note that three acceptable trials have been recorded, of which two trials have FVCs and FEV_1s that both agree within 5%.

CALCULATIONS

Most new pulmonary function equipment available today is equipped with a computer or microprocessor, which eliminates the need for manual calculation. However, manual calculation is required for the many manual volume-displacement spirometers still in use. Both the student and the technician should understand the basic calculations involved in order to use the manual devices when necessary and to better comprehend what the computer or microprocessor is doing.

The specific manual calculations vary with the volume-displacement spirometer and chart paper it uses. Spirometers designed with zero time-and-

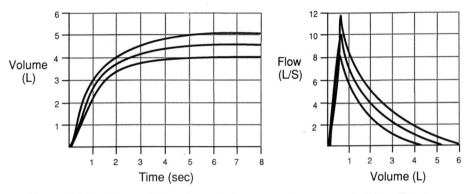

Figure 1.31. Unacceptable spirometry because of poor reproducibility. The two highest FVCs and two highest FEV₁s must agree within 5% or 100 ml, whichever is greater.

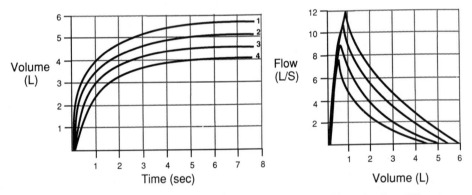

Figure 1.32. Forced spirometry on a patient who worsens with each effort. Effort 1 was done first, effort 2 second, etc.

volume starting points and supplied with temperature-corrected chart paper are the simplest and fastest to use. The calculations for spirometers that can rotate or operate at volumes other than zero and do not have temperature-corrected chart paper take longer, but results are considered to be more accurate. Before getting into these two different methods, it is important for the reader to first understand the issue of temperature correction.

Temperature Correction

When a patient blows into a spirometer tube, the exhaled air coming from the lungs is at 37°C and saturated with water vapor (BTPS). As this exhaled air travels toward the spirometer it cools. Charles' law states that the volume occupied by a given quantity of gas is directly related to temperature.

The gas exhaled into a volume-displacement spirometer will equilibrate at approximately the temperature of the spirometer (which is near room temperature). The gas exhaled into flow-sensing spirometers does not totally equilibrate until after it has passed out of the device, but it is generally accepted to be near room temperature.

Some time ago it was accepted that volumes measured during spirometry should be expressed as the volumes at body temperature. In order to convert volumes measured at room temperature (ATPS) to volumes at body temperature (BTPS), a factor must be applied. The formula for determining that factor is:

$$V(BTPS) = V(ATPS) \times \frac{PB - PH_2O}{PB - 47} \times \frac{310}{273 - Ta}$$

Where PB = barometric pressure in mm Hg; PH_2O = water vapor pressure at spirometer temperature; Ta = room (ambient) temperature; 47 = water vapor pressure at 37°C; 310 = absolute body temperature (Kelvin + 37, or 273 + 37); V(ATPS) = volume at ambient temperature and pressure saturated; V(BTPS) = volume at body temperature and pressure saturated.

The laboratory must be equipped to measure barometric pressure and temperature—either the temperature inside the spirometer or the room temperature near the spirometer. The temperature of the exhaled gas is equal to the room or spirometer temperature, PH_2O is taken from a chart, and the correction factor is calculated. When ATPS volumes are multiplied by this factor, BTPS volumes are obtained.

This method of correcting volumes is controversial. Can the spirometer temperature be equated with exhaled gas temperatures? Can the ATPS-to-BTPS factor be correctly applied to both volume-displacing spirometers and flow-sensing spirometers, and does room temperature accurately reflect spirometer temperature at the end of the FVC maneuver? These issues have been the subjects of several studies.[5-8]

Despite these concerns, temperature correction of spirometric values is still done in the manner described. The computerized devices make this correction automatically, some by assuming a barometric pressure and others by having the user enter a barometer reading.

To help the reader calculate the BTPS factor, Table 1.2 lists the water vapor pressures at various temperatures, which is needed for the formula above. Table 1.3 shows some common BTPS factors at two different altitudes.

Table 1.2: Water vapor pressure (PH₂O) at different temperatures

	Temperature	
	C	F	PH₂O
	20	68	18
	21	70	19
	22	72	20
	23	73	21
	24	75	22
	25	77	24
	26	79	25
	27	81	27

Table 1.3: Table corrections (ATPS to BTPS)

Room or Spirometer Temperature		ATPS to BTPS Factor at	
C	F	Sea Level	5000 Feet (PB = 625)
20	68	1.101	1.111
21	70	1.096	1.106
22	72	1.091	1.100
23	73	1.086	1.094
24	75	1.080	1.089
25	77	1.074	1.082
26	79	1.069	1.076
27	81	1.062	1.069

FVC and FEV₁ Measurement

First, let us deal with the spirometer with zero time-and-volume starting point that uses temperature-corrected chart paper. Figure 1.33 shows an example of three acceptable spirometry maneuvers starting from the zero time-and-volume point.

The largest FVC is easily identified. Note the reproducibility and good end-of-test technique. The largest FEV₁ is easily selected from the three volumes found on the 1-second line (the curves started exactly from the zero point). Values are read in liters at BTPS, but note that the chart paper states that BTPS correction is for 23°C. If the room or spirometer temperature varies by more than 2° from 23°, the BTPS correction may need to be recalculated. Differences of less than 2° will not matter clinically.

Calculation of FVC and FEV₁ from spirometers that have kymographs that can continually rotate or that operate at zero or other-than-zero volumes involves slightly more work, but the results are also more accu-

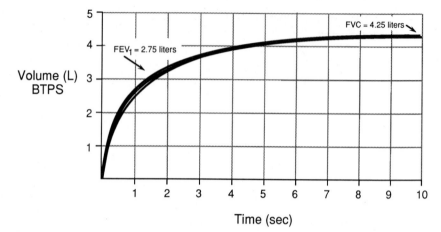

Figure 1.33. Acceptable spirometry as would be displayed in a volume-time format on chart paper frequently used on spirometers that are empty at the beginning of the test and that the pen always starts writing from the zero-time position. The FVC is read in liters on the volume axis at the highest pen deflection. The FEV_1 is read in liters on the volume axis where the pen deflection line crosses the 1-second line.

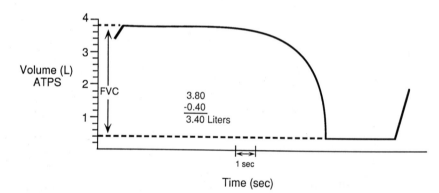

Figure 1.34. Forced spirometry maneuver as would be displayed in a volume-time format on chart paper frequently used on spirometers that rotate and are not necessarily empty at the beginning of the test (e.g., Stead-Wells water seal). The FVC is read in liters on the volume axis as the difference between the highest and lowest pen deflections.

rate. Usually the chart paper comes lined with ATPS volumes. When this is the case, measure the largest FVC by subtracting the starting volume from the ending volume as shown in Figure 1.34. The value is read in liters at ATPS with correction to BTPS to follow.

The largest FEV_1 is determined by using the **back extrapolation technique**. Because the FEV_1 is defined as the volume exhaled in the first

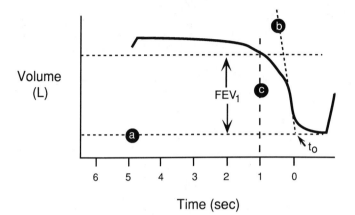

Time (sec)

Figure 1.35. Measurement of FEV$_1$ using the back extrapolation technique to define time-zero, or the point in the maneuver the patient started blowing as hard and as fast as possible. The technique requires a horizontal line at maximum inhalation "**a**," and a semivertical line passing through the steepest (most vertical) portion of the volume-time trace "**b**." The intersection of lines **a** and **b** becomes time-zero, from which time can be started and the true 1-second line drawn "**c**."

second of the FVC it is critical to identify the point from which time begins (i.e., the point when the patient started blowing as fast as possible). The back extrapolation technique, which helps define time-zero, is shown in Figure 1.35. The technician draws a line through the steepest portion of the forced expiratory curve. Where that line crosses the line drawn horizontally from maximum inhalation is the point known as time-zero (t_0). Once this point is known, measure 1 second over and then measure the volume for the FEV$_1$ in liters at ATPS. The extrapolated volume, shown in Figure 1.35, should not be greater than 5% of the FVC or 0.1 liter, whichever is greater. When it does exceed this limit, it is usually because of a poor start of test by the patient.

Once the FVC and FEV$_1$ have been corrected to BTPS, by determining the factor from the room or spirometer temperature and multiplying it by the volumes at ATPS, one can calculate one more value. It is the FEV$_1$ divided by the FVC and is sometimes referred to as the FEV$_1$/FVC ratio or FEV$_1$%. To calculate, simply divide the FEV$_1$ by the FVC and multiply by 100.

Other Spirometry Values

There are many values and measurements that can be calculated from the forced spirometry maneuver. It is not the intent of this chapter to demonstrate how each one is calculated by hand. Instead, it would seem appropriate to discuss the more commonly used measurements in terms of what they measure and their pitfalls.

The **FEF25-75%** is defined as the mean forced expiratory flow during the middle half of the FVC. In other words, it is the flow over the interval that starts after 25% of the FVC has been exhaled up to the point when 75% has been exhaled. It was originally described as the MMEF (maximal midexpiratory flow) and is reported in liters per second.[9] Many clinicians believe that it comes from a part of the spirogram that is relatively effort independent and that it describes the status of the small airways, which are thought to reflect early airway obstruction (earlier than other values such as FEV_1). For these reasons, FEF25-75% is frequently used to assess bronchodilator and provocation response. However, the FEF25-75% varies from test to test in patients with otherwise reproducible values and is very dependent on the size of the FVC. Some concern has existed about paradoxic responses of the FEF25-75% to bronchodilators. One study identified 21 out of 100 patients who had an improvement in FEV_1 but no improvement in the FEF25-75%.[10] When the investigators performed a volume adjustment technique (using the before-bronchodilator FVC to define the 25 and 75% points for the after-bronchodilator FEF25-75% measurement), 18 of the 21 patients showed improvement in FEF25-75%. The volume adjustment technique shown in Figure 1.36 merely transposes the 25 and 75% points from the before-drug curve to the after-drug curve. The resulting FEF25-75% is sometimes referred to as **isovolume FEF25-75%**.

In conjunction with the FEF25-75% is the **midexpiratory time (MET)**, also called the **forced expiratory time (FEF25-75%)**. Unlike the FEF25-75%, this measurement is the time (not flow) required to exhale the mid 50% of the expiratory curve. Because it is time, it is not dependent on the changes in the FVC as the FEF25-75% is and, therefore, does not need any corrections.

The flow volume curve or "loop" has become popular with the increased use of computerized spirometers. Graphic displays of flow and volume produce the best description of the mechanical properties of the lungs and, when plotted at absolute lung volume (i.e., the known total lung capacity obtained by first measuring FRC and then immediately performing the FVC maneuver), it is by far the best representation of pulmonary mechanics (Fig. 1.37).

The **peak expiratory flow rate (PEFR)**, also called the **maximal forced expiratory flow (FEFmax)** is the highest flow achieved during the FVC maneuver. It is not apparent from the conventional volume-time spirogram because it is an instantaneous flow. It is usually reported in liters

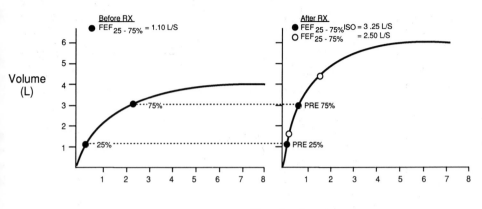

Time (sec)

Figure 1.36. Volume adjustment technique for calculating **isovolume FEF25-75%**. The FEF25-75% is calculated from a line connecting two points on the volume-time graph of the forced spirogram. One point is marked when 25% of the vital capacity has been exhaled; the other point is marked when 75% of the vital capacity has been exhaled. In the before-RX graph, the solid circles mark the 25 and 75% points. In the after-RX graph, the solid circles have been moved over from the before-RX graph (transposed) based on the before-RX volumes. The open circles mark the after-RX 25 and 75% points based on the after-RX volume. The **volume adjusted FEF25-75%** would be determined from a line connecting the solid circles on the after-RX graph—line **a**.

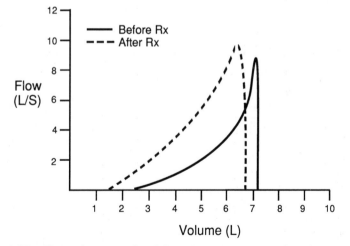

Volume (L)

Figure 1.37. Flow-volume graph of forced spirometry showing the measured curves before and after bronchodilator (RX). The placement of the curves is at absolute lung volumes arrived at by measuring FRC and immediately performing forced spirometry. Maximum inhalation level can be measured (FRC + inspiratory capacity) and used as the absolute volume level to place the curve.

per second. This parameter is a very effort-dependent value, and its poor reproducibility in a series of efforts should alert the technician to questionable efforts. Figure 1.38 shows two flow volume curves. Note the sharp point or peak with a good effort and the rounded pattern of a poor effort.

Figure 1.38 illustrates the **FEF25%, FEF50%,** and **FEF75%,** which are commonly reported expiratory flows. The 25, 50, and 75% modifiers refer to the amount of the FVC already exhaled. Like the FEFmax, these parameters are instantaneous flows and are usually reported in liters per second.

When a patient inspires as fast as possible after a forced expiration, a "loop" is formed. Figure 1.39 shows the flow volume loop with **FIF25%, FIF50%,** and **FIF75%.** The 25, 50 and 75% modifiers usually refer to the volume inspired from residual volume (RV).

A commonly reported ratio is the **FEF50%/FIF50%.** It is a comparison of midexpiratory flow to the midinspiratory flow. Normally, this ratio is between 0.8 and 1.2, which means that in normal individuals midexpiratory and midinspiratory flows are about the same. When this ratio is greater than 1.2, the inspiratory flow is low compared to the expiratory flow and can mean that the patient has an expiratory flow limitation.

The flow volume loop, as a picture, can be very informative. Figure 1.40 shows several flow volume loops that demonstrate different pulmonary function patterns. These patterns are easily identified by the trained eye without numbers or predicted values. For example, Figure 1.40A is a normal loop—note the straight downhill slope of the expiratory portion and the semicircle pattern of the inspiratory portion. Figure 1.40B has a scooped-out appearance on the expiratory portion, indicating airflow limitation. Figure 1.40C has a normal-looking expiratory portion, but the inspiratory flows are remarkably reduced. This type of pattern is seen in patients with a variable extrathoracic obstruction. Figure 1.40D has an abnormal-looking expiratory and inspiratory patern and is commonly seen in patients with a fixed airway obstruction. These observations are simplified but, nevertheless, demonstrate the usefulness of the loop.

Reporting of Results

After obtaining, calculating, or measuring three acceptable maneuvers, which values go onto the report? Usually, just one FVC, one FEV₁, and one of each of all the other values are reported. How does one choose? **The largest FVC and the largest FEV₁ (BTPS) should be reported, even if the two values come from different curves.**[2] Other measurements (e.g., FEF25-75%, or instantaneous flows) should be obtained from the sin-

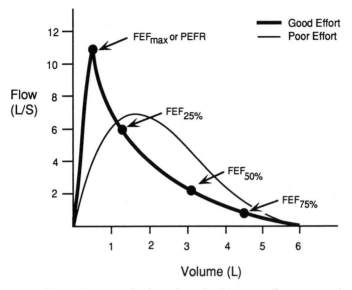

Figure 1.38. Flow-volume graph of two forced spirometry efforts—a good effort in the thick line, and a poor effort in the thin line. Note the difference in the peak flow pattern. The good effort contains solid circles that mark the FEFmax, FEF25% (the flow after 25% of the vital capacity has been exhaled), FEF50% (the flow after 50% of the vital capacity has been exhaled), and FEF75% (the flow after 75% of the vital capacity has been exhaled).

gle "best test" curve. The best test curve is that acceptable curve that has the largest sum of FVC and FEV_1, and some laboratories report even the FVC and FEV_1 from this curve (this was an acceptable method according to the 1979 ATS statement). Figure 1.41 shows three acceptable efforts on a volume-time display. Effort 1 has the largest FVC and effort 2 has the largest FEV_1. The best test curve (the curve with the largest sum of FVC and FEV_1) is effort 2 and thus is the curve from which the FEF25-75% should be taken.

All results should be expressed in liters at BTPS, rounded to two decimal points.

REFERENCE VALUES

It is a common practice to compare each measured or calculated variable in a patient's pulmonary function study to a reference or predicted value. This comparison provides a basis for interpreting the patient's values. A complete listing of reference values is in Appendix 4.

Studies designed to establish "normal" or reference values are large undertakings. An investigator must first choose and define a population

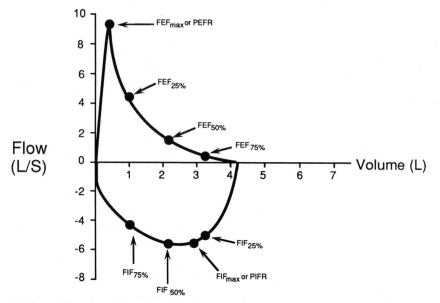

Figure 1.39. Flow-volume graph of forced spirometry with inspiratory and expiratory portions completing a "loop." The inspiratory portion contains solid circles marking commonly measured points—FIF25% (forced inspiratory flow after 25% of the vital capacity has been inhaled from residual volume or maximum expiratory level), FIF50% (forced inspiratory flow after 50% of the vital capacity has been inhaled), FIF75% (forced inspiratory flow after 75% of the vital capacity has been inhaled), and FIFmax (maximum inspiratory flow, also known as peak inspiratory flow rate).

(e.g., urban boys age 6 to 12) and, by means of a detailed questionnaire, find subjects who are nonsmokers (or those who have never smoked) and who do not have any present or past acute or chronic respiratory problems (such as shortness of breath, cough, or wheezing). Next, these healthy subjects are given pulmonary function tests, and their results make up the reference or "normal" values. Of course, enough healthy subjects of the specified age and sex must be tested to make the study useful.

The study of a well-defined, healthy population results in reference values in the form of an interval. This interval or range of "normal" values represents usually 95% of the sample population for different sex, height, age, and weight. If we performed pulmonary function tests on 100 normal men, each 30 years old, 68 inches (173 cm), and weighing 160 lb (73 kg), most would have different measured values for each pulmonary function parameter. The different values would be scattered around the mean for each parameter. This scattering is shown in Figure 1.42 and is referred to as a normal frequency distribution. Notice the clustering in the middle, creat-

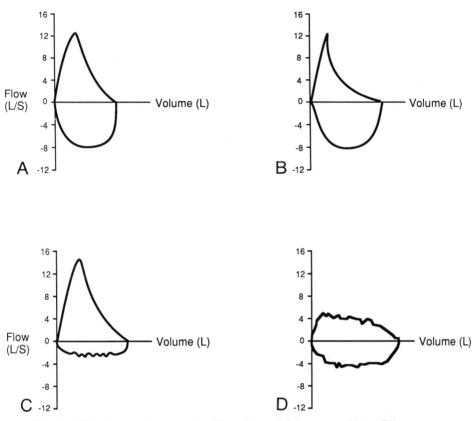

Figure 1.40. Flow-volume graphs of four "loops." **A** is a normal loop. **B** has a normal inspiratory portion, but the expiratory portion is "scooped-out," which is commonly seen in patients with airflow limitation (e.g., asthma or emphysema). **C** has a reduced inspiratory portion and a normal expiratory portion. This usually suggests an obstruction that is above the thoracic cage (e.g., larynx) that limits inspiratory flow rate. **D** has reduced inspiratory and expiratory portions, a characteristic that is commonly seen in patients with a fixed airway obstruction.

ing a bell-shape pattern. The width of a normal distribution is described by its standard deviation (S) and the average by its mean. Figure 1.42 also shows that 95% of the points are within approximately ± 2 S (exactly 1.96 S).

When interpreting spirometric results, the concern is to identify the lower limit of "normal." One method is to use the 95% confidence interval for each parameter. This is usually reported in the reference study or can be calculated from the equation:

95% confidence interval = mean value ± 1.64 standard deviations

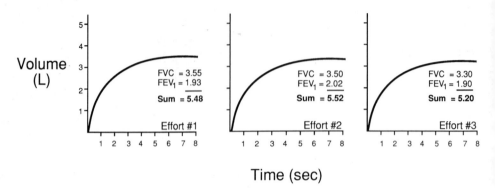

Figure 1.41. Volume-time graph of three acceptable forced spirometry efforts. Effort 1 has the highest FVC (3.55 liters), and effort 2 has the highest FEV₁ (2.02 liters). Effort 2 also has the highest sum of FVC and FEV₁ and would thus be called the "best curve."

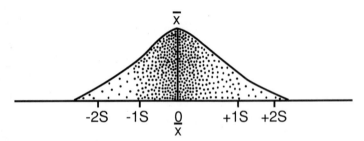

Figure 1.42. Frequency distribution of a pulmonary function parameter on 100 normal men with the same age and height. Of the 100 values obtained, many are the same and are clustered in the center, with fewer value points scattered to the sides, creating a bell-shape pattern of normal distribution. The width of this normal distribution is described by its standard deviation (S)—95% of the points are within the boundaries of ±2 standard deviations, and 90% are within ±1 standard deviation.

Another commonly used method is to use 80% of the predicted value as the lower limit of normal. However, this method has shortcomings because using 80% of the predicted value as the lower limit of "normal" cannot be applied to all values. For example, the lower limit of normal for the FEF25-75% would probably be closer to 70% of the predicted value.

The factors most affecting pulmonary function test values have been determined from observation and analysis of results of testing large groups of "normals" and include age, height, sex, and race. Spirometry values such as FVC and FEV₁ increase throughout childhood and plateau between the ages of 20 and 30 years. After that age, these values decline. Taller people and men have bigger lung volumes. Lung volumes for non-Caucasians are lower than lung volumes for Caucasians of the same age, height, and sex. The explanation is that there are differences in thoracic cage size and diaphragm position. Using Caucasian reference values with a non-Caucasian patient may produce a falsely low percent of predicted value.

The use of reference values has raised some concerns including the following: (*a*) there are not enough values for certain races and age groups (e.g., those over 70 years); (*b*) a patient may be called "normal" when compared to one set of reference values but "abnormal" when compared to another set because of variability among the reference studies; (*c*) different types of equipment have been used to measure the subjects, which might contribute to the differences between studies; (*d*) there are many studies available to choose from, but not all of them contain all of the pulmonary function values; therefore, some laboratories are forced to mix reference values from different studies; (*e*) older studies sometimes included ex-smokers and even current smokers in their sample. These and other concerns have been raised, but as yet, there is no universally accepted set of reference values. However, a recent survey found that most pulmonary teaching programs rely on information in only a few studies.[11]

Suggestions when selecting reference values for a laboratory

a. Choose from published studies.
b. Choose studies that use the same race as the patient.
c. Choose studies that use similar equipment.
d. Check the reference values against a sample of normals in the laboratory by testing 5 to 10 individuals who are nonsmokers and who do not have respiratory problems. The pulmonary function results of the laboratory "normals" should produce values that are within the confidence intervals of the reference study. If not the reference values used may not "fit" the population that will be tested in the laboratory, and other reference values should be considered.

Once a selection has been made, the common method is to compare the observed patient data to the mean reference value. **The percent of predicted value** is determined by dividing the observed value by the reference value, and the resulting decimal is multiplied by 100.

Some computerized spirometers offer the user a choice of reference values. The documentation accompanying the spirometer usually provides the names of the primary investigators and the date the study was performed (e.g., Crapo 1981). But no description of the equipment used or the racial makeup of the population is provided. Appendix 4 supplies a description of equipment used and the racial makeup of the study sample for commonly used reference values.

Some spirometer systems offer a "racial correction" factor—the reduction of selected reference values by a fixed percentage (often 15%), but, in some systems, a choice of percentages is offered. However, the differences among ethnic groups can be too variable to be corrected by the application of a constant scaling factor for all pulmonary function parameters. It is most desirable to use reference values derived from a sample of the ethnic group to which the subject belongs. However, if such reference values are not available, an alternative is to use reference values from a Caucasian population and allow for differences in the interpretation.

When a patient is seen for the first time, the pulmonary function test results are usually compared to reference equations for interpretation. Although this comparison is not a good diagnostic tool, it may be useful to exclude disease. Because a patient's FEV_1 falls below the lower limit of the confidence interval does not mean it could not be "normal" in another reference study of another sample population. Therefore, when using reference values, use them as one part of the diagnostic process.

Another approach is to observe and compare changes in the patient over time (a longitudinal study). Sequential tests at 6 months or a year, for example, can determine whether a patient's function is worsening, improving, or not changing—except for aging. The expected decrease in FVC and FEV_1 from aging is approximately 25 to 30 ml per year. Figure 1.43 demonstrates why observing and comparing changes in a patient over time can be more valuable than simple comparison of results to a reference value. Figure 1.43A shows two patients on a graph of a pulmonary function value reference equation. The regression line of the equation slopes downward (declines) with age, and the shaded area represents the 95% confidence interval. Patient 1 is above the regression line, in fact above the 95% confidence interval, and would be called supranormal. Patient 2, however, is below the 95% level and would be called abnormal. Figure 1.43B shows the same two patients measured again 2 years later. Patient 2 is still below the 95% level and would be still called "abnormal" but is declining at the expected normal rate (25 to 30 ml/year). However, although patient 1 is still normal, he/she is declining at a rate much faster than would be expected and is the patient about whom we should be concerned. One might say that following the change in percent-predicted values would reveal the

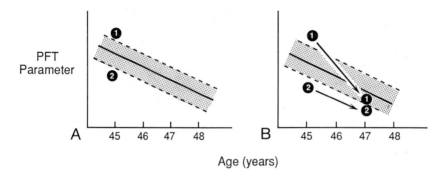

Age (years)

Figure 1.43. Pulmonary function test (PFT) results and reference regression line (*solid*) with the 95% confidence intervals (*dashed*) on two patients (1 and 2). **A** shows they were both tested at 45 years of age. Patient 1 is above the 95% confidence interval for this particular parameter and would be called normal or even above-normal. Patient 2 falls below the 95% confidence interval and would be called abnormal. **B** shows both patients measured again at age 47. Patient 2 is still below the 95% confidence interval and would again be called abnormal. Patient 1 is within the 95% confidence interval and would be called normal. However, patient 1 is declining faster than the reference regression line and faster than patient 2 and thus is the patient about whom we should be concerned.

same information; however, the same predicted values are not always used, and in many laboratories the predicted values are not noted on pulmonary function reports.

BRONCHODILATORS

Frequently in the pulmonary function laboratory or office, bronchodilators are given to determine whether airflow limitation is reversible. A patient does not have to be "obstructed," wheeze, or complain of shortness of breath to indicate the use of bronchodilators. Bronchodilator administration can be built into the spirometry procedure or may be indicated when suspicion of asthma persists despite "normal" spirometry results.

Medications that reduce bronchospasm or airflow obstruction are called bronchodilators. Many such medications are available for administration by inhalation, orally, intramuscularly, or intravenously. The discussion in this section will focus on the aerosolized medications because they are used most commonly in the pulmonary function laboratory.

Bronchodilators increase airway caliber by relaxing airway smooth muscle. The aerosolized bronchodilators are usually sympathomimetic (adrenergic) and affect the two primary types of adrenergic receptors located in the bronchial smooth muscle and blood vessels—α and β. The α-receptors cause vasoconstriction. The β-receptors, which can be divided into two groups (β-1 and β-2) cause vasodilation, bronchodilation, and increased heart rate—among other things. The β-1 receptors increase heart rate more than they dilate bronchi, and the β-2 receptors cause more bronchodilation than increased heart rate.

There are several aerosolized bronchodilators that are commonly used in the pulmonary function laboratory. One is **isoproterenol**, which is fast acting (peak effect occurs within 5 to 10 minutes), but which is also short lasting (its effects usually last less than 2 hours). The major complaint of using isoproterenol is that it has a strong β-1 action, so large increases in heart rate are commonly noted.

Another commonly used medication is **metaproterenol**, which is primarily a β-2 stimulator, but it can cause increased heart rate. Like other primarily β-2 (e.g., **albuterol** and **terbutaline**) drugs, the peak effect is slower (15 to 30 minutes), and the duration of action is longer lasting.

Which bronchodilator and how much of it to administer is a decision usually made by the ordering physician. However, many laboratories have a written procedure for bronchodilator administration (including type and amount) if the physician has not specified such information.

Aerosolized bronchodilators can be given in several ways: (*a*) metered dose inhalers (MDI); (*b*) jet nebulizers powered by compressed air; and (*c*) nebulizers powered by hand-squeezed bulbs. Administration by a nebulizer incorporated into an intermittent positive pressure breathing (IPPB) system was more popular in the 1970s and early 1980s but is infrequently used today.

Studies suggest that an appropriate and effective dose of bronchodilator can be administered as effectively by MDI as by a nebulizer. However, the addition of a spacer can increase the effectiveness in some patients. The spacer acts as a reservoir from which the patient breathes the medication, reducing the importance of timing the actuation of the MDI unit. Another alternative to the reservoir type spacer is an extension of tubing between the MDI and the mouth. This extension acts to trap larger particles so that less medication is deposited in the mouth and larynx.

The method for using an MDI is important. The technician should supervise if not perform the actuation of the MDI. The procedure is not standardized but should include (*a*) slowly exhaling to near RV; (*b*) having the patient slowly inhale, activating the MDI just after the inhalation starts; (*c*) having the patient continue to inhale slowly as deeply as possible; (*d*) having the patient hold his/her breath for 2 to 5 seconds and slowly exhale; and (*e*) waiting 30 to 60 seconds and repeating with a second inhalation.

In some laboratories, more than two actuations of a MDI (a common clinical dose) is administered. In these laboratories the actuations continue until side effects are achieved (e.g., increased heart rate, shakiness, or headache). The reason for more than two actuations is to ensure that the patient has gotten a "good" treatment, which is indicated by the side effects. If a laboratory is considering such a method, a protocol should be written describing the contraindications and side effect limits.

After the administration of the bronchodilator, the technician should wait at least 5 to 10 minutes before repeating the pulmonary function tests. This will ensure that the medication is approaching or is at peak effect.

Summary of key points in bronchodilator administration in the PF lab

---

1. *Use an appropriate bronchodilator—one ordered by the physician, used clinically by the patient, or one specified in the laboratory procedure manual.*
2. *Administer or supervise patient administration of the ordered amount or an amount that is clinically useful, with the nebulizer and/or spacer.*
3. *Wait an appropriate amount of time before repeating pulmonary tests.*
4. *Note amount and method of administration in comments.*

Reporting Bronchodilator Therapy

The pulmonary function report should include a list of the pulmonary medications the patient took prior to and during the test. The laboratory treatment should state which drug (generic name) and how much was given (e.g., two puffs—metered dose inhaler). In order to report medications taken prior to testing, the technician must ask the patient. Because there are numerous medications and combinations of medications it is important for the technician to know the mode of action, route of administration, and generic versus trade name. Additionally, because taking certain medications prior to a pulmonary function test may contraindicate performing the test, the duration of action should also be known. Therefore, I have included a listing of drugs frequently used by patients with pulmonary disease. Table 1.4 lists these drugs by both generic and trade names, route of administration, and duration of action.

Table 1.4: Medications frequently taken by patients being tested in the pulmonary function laboratory listed by generic name, trade name, route of administration, and duration of action (in hours)

Generic Name	Trade Name	Route	Duration of Action (hours)
Terbutaline	Brethine	Oral	4–8
		Subcutaneous	1.5–4
	Bricanyl	Oral	4–8
		Subcutaneous	1.5–4
	Brethaire	MDI	4–6
Albuterol	Proventil	Oral	4–6
		Sol,MDI	4–6
	Ventolin	Oral	4–6
		Sol,MDI	4–6
Metaproterenol	Alupent	Oral	4
		Sol,MDI	3–4
	Metaprel	Oral	4
		Sol,MDI	3–4
Isoetharine	Bronkosol	Sol	1–3
	Bronkometer	MDI	1–3
Isoproterenol	Isuprel	Sol,MDI	0.5–2
	Aerolone	Sol,MDI	0.5–2
Rac epinephrine	Vaponefrin	Sol	1–3
Epinephrine	Primatine Mist	MDI	?
	Bronitin Mist	MDI	?
	Adrenaline	IM, Subcutaneous	<1–4
Ephedrine	Ephedrine	IM, Subcutaneous, IV	10–20 min
Bitolterol	Tornulate	MDI	5–8
Atropine	Atropine	Sol	<1–4
Ipratropium	Atrovent	MDI	>4
Cromolyn sodium	Intal	Sol, MDI	
Beclamethasone	Beclovent	MDI	
	Vanceril	MDI	
Dexamethasone	Respihaler	MDI	
Triamcinolone	Azmacort	MDI	
Flunisolide	Aerobid	MDI	
Prednisone	Many	Oral	
Theophylline	Many	Oral	

INTERPRETATION

The pulmonologist is usually responsible for interpreting the results of pulmonary function tests. However, it is helpful for the technician to know the basics of spirometric interpretation because it helps him/her to collect better and more useful information and to better understand the patient's condition and the changes that occur.

The forced spirogram provides information about the flow and volume of air moving in and out of the lungs in one rapid inhalation and forced expiration. When the airways are narrowed, the flow through them will be reduced. The narrowing of the airways can result from bronchospasm (smooth muscle contraction), inflammation, increased mucus, tumors (either internal or external to the airway), or loss of elasticity, resulting in airway collapse. This reduction in airflow is referred to as **airflow limitation**. An older and less precise term used to describe the reduced airflow is "obstruction" as in "airway obstruction" and "obstructive airway disease." However, it implies that the reduction in airflow is from material inside the airway, which is only one of many reasons for airway narrowing.

Many parameters can be measured from the forced spirogram or flow-volume loop, but only a few are helpful in the interpretation process. Specifically, this section will address the FVC, FEV_1, and the FEV_1/FVC ratio.

The FVC is the maximum volume of air exhaled after a maximum inhalation. A FVC below the limits of normal—even though effort was maximal—can be due to (a) airflow limitation wherein air is trapped in the alveoli due to collapsing airways and/or causes a reduced driving force due to decreased elasticity, or (b) reduced lung size caused by a restrictive process (e.g., interstitial lung disease, neuromuscular disease, or chest wall disorders).

The FEV_1 is the volume exhaled in the first second of the FVC. It too can be reduced because of airflow limitation and a restrictive process.

The ratio of FEV_1/FVC (usually multiplied by 100 and expressed as a percent) distinguishes between airflow limitation and a restrictive process as the basis for the reduction in FEV_1 and FVC. In patients with airflow limitation, the FEV_1/FVC ratio (also called $FEV_1\%$) is reduced, but, in patients with restrictive disease, the ratio is normal or increased. This ratio, however, is not very useful in measuring response to bronchodilator in patients with airflow limitation because the FVC may also change. Table 1.5 compares the spirometric data of two patients—one with airflow limitation, the other with a restrictive process. It can be seen that the FEV_1/FVC ratio clearly distinguishes the patient with airflow limitation from the patient with a restrictive process. It can also be seen that the patient with airflow limitation responds to bronchodilator (23% improvement in FEV_1 and 18% improvement in FVC), but the FEV_1/FVC ratio does not change significantly.

Additionally, there can be a mixed obstructive and restrictive disease process that is very difficult to confirm with spirometry alone. The measurements of functional residual capacity, residual volume, and total lung capacity must also be made.

Table 1.5: Examples of data from forced spirometry on two patients before and after bronchodilator[a]

	Predicted Value	Airflow Limitation Before	Airflow Limitation After	Restrictive Process Before	Restrictive Process After
FVC (L)	4.70	2.93 (62)[b]	3.46 (74)	2.93 (62)	2.95 (63)
FEV$_1$ (L)	3.56	1.29 (34)	1.59 (45)	2.63 (74)	2.69 (76)
FEV$_1$/FVC (%)	76	44	46	90	91

[a]One patient has airflow limitation, and the second patient has a restrictive process. The reference values are obtained from the standards of Morris (Morris JF, Koski A, Johnson LC. Spirometric standards for healthy nonsmoking adults. Am Rev Respir Dis 1971; 103: 57–67) using a male, 68 inches tall, and 45 years old.
[b]Values in parentheses are percent of predicted.

The interpretation of the forced spirogram will vary depending on the interpreter. Some interpreters will only make an observation such as "airflow limitation" or "reduced FEV$_1$," but others will quantify the observations by stating "moderate airflow limitation" or "moderately reduced FEV$_1$." There is no agreement on what is mild, moderate, or severe. I use the following guide to interpret the forced spirogram with an inspiratory loop.

Interpretation of Bronchodilator Response

The interpretation of the effect of a bronchodilator drug is focused on change in certain pulmonary function parameters. In healthy individuals, the FVC increases approximately 11%, the FEV$_1$ increases approximately 8%, and the FEF50% increases approximately 17%.[12] Additionally, the FEV$_1$ appears to be the best indicator of responsiveness to bronchodilator in a general population sample.[12] However, the response in patients with lung disease is much greater. The American College of Chest Physicians recommends an increase of 15 to 25% in at least two or three spirometric tests (FVC, FEV$_1$, and FEF25-75%).[13] Another recommendation is to call an increase in FEV$_1$ of 15%, and 30% in the FEF25-75% (measured at isovolume) clinically significant.[14] A similar recommendation (i.e., FEV$_1$ of 12.3% and FEF25-75% of 45.1%) was made in a study[15] that used 95% confidence intervals of percent change to evaluate change.

SPECIAL CONSIDERATIONS

Obtaining acceptable spirometry results is not an easy task. A number of patient, technician, and equipment constraints must be satisfied. What happens when the patient is not cooperative, is unable to follow directions, or is physically unable to do what is asked? When such problems occur, the

For the forced expiratory curve:

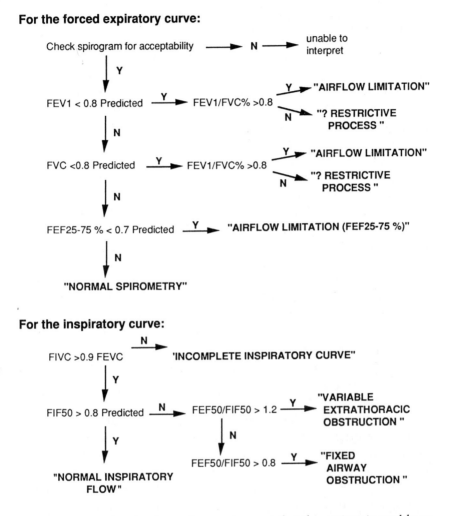

For the inspiratory curve:

technician may dismiss the patient and report that the patient is unable to perform spirometry. However, in many of these instances, spirometry can be adequately performed if the technician is skilled and patient.

Most patients come to the hospital or office because they are sincerely seeking help. They are willing to do most things that they are asked and are cooperative. A small percentage of patients are not willing to try doing what is asked of them and are not very cooperative. Sometimes such patients are involved in legal actions, and gain or loss may ride on the test outcome. What does one say to these uncooperative patients? How does one get them to do an effort-dependent test like spirometry? One technique is to have the ordering physician give the patient a "pep talk," stressing the importance of trying as hard as possible. Another technique is for the technician to tell the uncooperative patient that "the data obtained thus far are not reportable, and therefore, the physicians (and/or litigation system) cannot proceed." This direct, no-nonsense approach frequently works with uncooperative patients.

Some patients have difficulty following directions, for example, the very young, the very old, and the hearing impaired. Young children often do better with their parents close by helping with instructions, coaching, and discipline. Occasionally, however, a child performs better when the parent is not around. The young child's short attention span and inability to sit quietly for the necessary length of time make pulmonary function testing difficult, and a skilled technician who can work quickly and efficiently is required. Many trials may be needed. One recommendation is to do a minimum of five and a maximum of eight FVC maneuvers to obtain at least three acceptable efforts.[16]

The very old may have many problems (e.g., poor coordination, hearing impairment, fatigue, illness, etc.). The key to successful pulmonary function testing in these patients is patience. The technician needs to explain the instructions for the procedure carefully, repeat as frequently as the circumstances dictate, and be prepared and willing to take extra time.

The hearing impaired and those who do not speak English need to hear and understand what the technician wants them to do. An interpreter should be provided to relay instructions in sign language or the subject's native language. For those who wear hearing aids and still do not hear well or for those who just don't hear well enough to catch all of the details, written instructions may work well. Hearing aids amplify all sounds and, in noisy environments, discriminating the speech sounds from the other sounds may be a problem. Because most hearing impaired people lip-read very well, the technician should speak slowly and clearly while looking directly at the patient. Again, patience is the key to success.

Another group of patients who need special considerations are those who are physically unable to perform the test in the standard manner—for example, patients with tracheostomies or patients who cannot seal the mouthpiece tightly because of a paralysis or malformation of the lips or mouth. Ingenuity is the key to successfully working with such patients. For example, an infant positive-pressure mask connected to the spirometer via a tubing adapter can be fitted over the tracheal stoma.

INFECTION CONTROL

The role of respiratory therapy equipment in nosocomial infections usually receives great attention. However, the role of pulmonary function equipment in the transmission of infections is often ignored and has not been established.

Microorganisms reportedly have been collected from pulmonary function devices.[17,18] The transmission of the microorganisms to other patients and technicians has also been reported.[19]

It is probably safe to speculate that there is a risk of cross-contamination when using pulmonary function equipment. It would also seem safe to speculate that this risk is inversely proportional to the frequency of cleaning or changing equipment parts. The use of filters to trap microorganisms might reduce this risk, however filter use is costly and may interfere with accuracy.

My recommendations are:

1. Use disposable mouthpieces and discard after single patient use. If using rubber mouthpieces, change between patients and clean with high-level disinfection (inactivation of vegetative microorganisms but not necessarily bacterial spores).
2. External spirometer tubing should be changed between patients. The contaminated tubing should receive high-level disinfection and be dried before reuse.
3. Noseclips should be changed between patients and discarded or cleaned with high-level disinfection.
4. Change water in water-sealed spirometers monthly.
5. Don't spend a great amount of time and effort cleaning the surfaces inside the spirometers.[18]
6. Wash hands thoroughly using good handwashing technique before and after performing pulmonary function testing procedures whether or not gloves are worn.

CASE 1.1

A 16-year-old boy was tested in the pulmonary function laboratory. The ordering doctor noted that the diagnosis was asthma. The results of each spirometry trial are shown in Table 1.6 and Figure 1.44.

Questions
1. What is the interpretation/evaluation of these spirometric tests?
2. Which before and after efforts should be reported?

Answers and Discussion
The first FVC effort (9:05) shows mild airflow limitation based on the reduced FEV_1/FVC% and FEF25-75% (43% of predicted value). The remaining before-RX efforts show significant deterioration.

The after-RX forced expiratory efforts show marked improvement in airflow. The amount of improvement is dependent on which before-RX effort is used for comparison.

Table 1.6: Spirometric results of each trial before and after bronchodilator (RX) on 16-year-old male in Case 1.1

	Time	FVC(L)	FEV$_1$ FEV$_1$(L)	FEF 25–75% FVC(%)	(L/S)
Before RX					
FVC 1	9:05	4.13	3.01	73	2.03
FVC 2	9:07	3.61	2.48	69	1.63
FVC 3	9:08	3.42	2.41	70	1.69
FVC 4	9:10	3.12	2.01	64	1.48
FVC 5	9.12	3.09	2.02	65	1.51
After RX					
FVC 1	9:40	4.33	3.30	76	2.59
FVC 2	9.42	4.29	3.31	77	2.63
FVC 3	9.43	4.32	3.33	77	2.58

The deterioration of flow rates in the before-RX test could be caused by poor effort or spirometry-induced bronchoconstriction. Poor effort is a factor that should be assessed by the technician. The diagnosis of asthma makes the likely cause the spirometry itself.

The effects of deep inspiration have been studied and have shown varying effects on airflow. In some asthmatics, a deep inspiration causes bronchoconstriction that comes on rapidly and may disappear spontaneously in a minute or two.[20-22] In nonasthmatics a deep inspiration has been shown to cause a bronchodilating effect.[23]

Traditionally one before-bronchodilator and one after-bronchodilator effort is reported. In Case 1.1, if the first before-RX effort is selected (based on highest values) the comparison to after-RX efforts would show only a small improvement. However, if the fifth before-RX effort is selected, which best represents the patient's airflow before the bronchodilator, the interpretation is quite different. Alternatively, both the first and fifth efforts could be reported to show the deterioration, or a comment could be made noting the deterioration.

CASE 1.2

A 42-year-old white female was seen in the pulmonary function laboratory. The ordering doctor had noted asthma as the diagnosis and that she was being treated with theophylline and inhaled bronchodilators. The results from her pulmonary function tests are shown in Table 1.7.

Questions
1. What is the interpretation/evaluation of these spirometric tests?

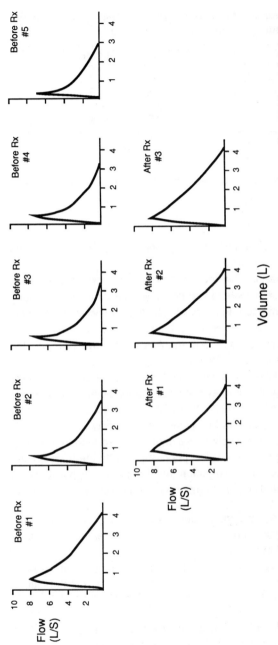

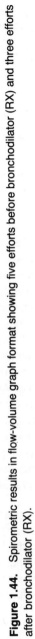

Figure 1.44. Spirometric results in flow-volume graph format showing five efforts before bronchodilator (RX) and three efforts after bronchodilator (RX).

Table 1.7: Pulmonary function results before and after bronchodilator (two actuations of metaproterenol metered dose inhaler)

	Before	After	% Change
FVC (L)	2.90 (89)*	3.00	3
FEV$_1$ (L)	2.02 (74)	2.18	8
FEV$_1$/FVC (%)	70	73	
FEF25–75% (L/S)	2.41 (74)	2.62	9

*Values in parentheses are percent of predicted.

2. What issues would be raised with these results, given the diagnosis and medication regimen?

Answers and Discussion

The spirometry data reveal airflow limitation with only minimal response to the two "puffs" of the metaproterenol MDI.

One question to be asked is whether or not bronchodilators were withheld prior to this spirometric test. A bronchodilator taken within 8 hours of spirometry can affect results and interpretation. Inhaled bronchodilators should be withheld for their duration of action (usually 4 to 8 hours) prior to such a test. The advisability of withholding oral theophylline and β-agonists is controversial, and the directive of the physician should be followed.

Another question is whether the patient has hyperreactive airways that respond to bronchodilators. If not, she may not need the medications with which she is being treated. A bronchial provocation test (e.g., methacholine) would determine the presence or absence of bronchial hyperreactivity (asthma).

In this particular case, a methacholine challenge revealed moderate airway hyperreactivity, which is surprising given her poor response to the bronchodilator during spirometry. However, there are a number of reasons why patients with hyperreactive airways (asthma) may not respond to bronchodilators:

1. The medication is trapped in the mouth and does not reach the airways.
2. The large airways are physically narrowed, resulting in decreased amounts of medication reaching the lower airways.
3. The patient has a bronchospastic reaction to the propellent used in the MDI.
4. The patient has problems with techniques (e.g., coordination, breathholding, and/or rate of inhalation).

It is possible that, in this patient, any or several of these reasons played a role. Although the usual clinical dose from a MDI is two actuations, it may be necessary to deliver more to demonstrate bronchodilator improvement.

The spirometry was repeated several days later. This time, however, the order was for six actuations unless the patient developed side effects (e.g.,

Table 1.8: Pulmonary function results before and after bronchodilator (six actuations of metaproterenol MDI)

	Before	After	% Change
FVC (L)	2.83	3.19	13
FEV$_1$ (L)	1.98	2.47	25
FEV$_1$/FVC (%)	70	77	
FEF25–75% (L/S)	2.46	3.39	38

tremors, tachycardia, palpitation, headache). The results are shown in Table 1.8.

These results clearly show that this patient responds to the bronchodilator, which is consistent with the methacholine challenge. In this case, six actuations were enough and, possibly, four or five would also be enough. The usual dose of two actuations has been established as the dose that usually does not cause side effects and usually results in improvement. But, in some patients more actuations are required.

REFERENCES

1. American Thoracic Society Statement. Standardization of spirometry. Am Rev Respir Dis 1979;119:831–838.
2. American Thoracic Society Statement. Standardization of spirometry. Am Rev Respir Dis 1987;136:1030–1050.
3. Nelson SB, Gardner RM, Crapo RO, Jensen RL. Performance evaluation of contemporary spirometers. Chest 1990;97:288–297.
4. Hepper NGG, Black LF, Fowler WS. Relationships of lung volumes to height and arm span in normal subjects and in patients with spinal deformity. Am Rev Respir Dis 1965;91:356–362.
5. Tashkin DP, Patel A, Calverese B, et al. Overestimation of forced expiratory volumes and flow rates measured by volumetric spirometry when ATPS to BTPS correction is applied [abstract]. Am Rev Respir Dis 1981;123:83.
6. Tashkin DP, Patel A, Deutsch R, et al. Is standard ATPS to BTPS correction of volumes and flow rates measured with a volumetric spirometer valid? [Abstract]. Am Rev Respir Dis 1980;121:412.
7. Pincock AC, Miller MR. The effect of temperature on recording spirograms. Am Rev Respir Dis 1983;128:894–898.
8. Hankenson JL, Viola JO. Dynamic BTPS correction factors for spirometric data. J Appl Physiol 1983;55:1354–1360.
9. Leuallen EC, Fowler WS. Maximal midexpiratory flow. Am Rev Tuberc 1955;72:783–800.
10. Cockcroft DW, Bersheid BA. Volume adjustment to maximal midexpiratory flow. Chest 1980;4:595–600.
11. Ghio AJ, Crapo RO, Elliot CG. Reference equations used to predict pulmonary function. Chest 1990;97:400–403.
12. Lorber DB, Kaltenborn W, Burrows B. Responses to isoproterenol in a general sample. Am Rev Respir Dis 1978;118:885–861.
13. Committee on Emphysema-ACCP, G Synider Chairman. Criteria for the assessment of reversibility of airway obstruction. Chest 1974;65:552–553.
14. Clausen JL, ed. Pulmonary function testing. Guidelines and controversies. New York: Academic Press, 1982:215–221.
15. Sourk RL, Nugent KM. Bronchodilator testing: Confidence intervals derived from placebo inhalations. Am Rev Respir Dis 1983;128:153–157.

16. Kanner RE, Schenker MB, Munoz A, Speizer FE. Spirometry in children. Am Rev Respir Dis 1983;127:720–724.

17. Tablan OC, Williams WW, Martone WJ. Infection control in pulmonary function laboratories. Infect Control 1985;6:442–444.

18. Rutala DR, Rutala WA, Weber DJ, Thomann CA. Infection risks associated with spirometry. Infect Control Hosp Epidemiol 1991;12:89–92.

19. Hazaleus RE, Cole J, Berdischewsky M. Tuberculin skin test conversion from exposure to contaminated pulmonary function testing apparatus. Resp Care 1981;26:53–55.

20. Gayrard P, Orekek J, Grimaud C, Charpin J. Bronchoconstrictor effects of a deep inspiration in patients with asthma. ARRD 1975;111:433–439.

21. Lloyd TC. Bronchoconstriction in man following single deep inspirations. J Appl Physiol 1963;18:114–116.

22. Mackay AD, Mustchin CP, Sterling GM. The response of asthmatic patients and normal subjects to maximum respiratory maneuvers [Supplement]. Eur J Respir Dis 1980;61:35–40.

23. Nadel JA, Tierney DA. Effect of a previous deep inspiration on airway resistance in man. J Appl Physiol 1961;16:717–719.

SELF-ASSESSMENT QUESTIONS

1. During a forced expiration, the point in the airways where the pleural pressure equals the airway pressure is called the:

   a. equal airway pressure
   b. null pressure point
   c. equal pressure point
   d. transpulmonary pressure

2. All of the following are examples of a volume-displacement spirometer except:

   a. water-seal
   b. bellows
   c. balloon
   d. rolling-seal

3. All of the following are examples of flow-sensing spirometers except:

   a. pneumotach
   b. thermistor
   c. wedge
   d. vortex

4. Calibration of spirometers should be done with a good quality syringe of known volume:

   a. before every patient
   b. every day it is used
   c. once per week
   d. once per month

5. All of the following are acceptability criteria for spirometric maneuvers except:
   a. no coughing
   b. no early termination
   c. good reproducibility of efforts
   d. good start of test
   e. none of above

6. When calibrating a spirometer with a known-volume calibration syringe, the volume measured should be within what percentage of the known volume?
   a. ± 1%
   b. ± 3%
   c. ± 5%
   d. ± 7%

7. Spirometric values are reported as the amount at:
   a. ATPS
   b. BTPS
   c. STPD
   d. ATPD

8. Several concerns have been raised about the use of reference values. Which of the following is not a concern?
   a. not enough values for certain races and age groups
   b. use of different types of instrumentation
   c. inclusion of current and exsmokers in some studies
   d. not all values are contained in one study
   e. none of above

9. Which of the following medications is not used in the pulmonary function laboratory as a bronchodilator?
   a. metaproterenol
   b. albuterol
   c. cromolyn sodium
   d. isoproterenol

10. According to the 1987 ATS Standards Statement, the acceptable limit for back extrapolated volume as a percent of the vital capacity is less than:
   a. 10%
   b. 7%
   c. 5%
   d. 3%

2

Lung Volumes

The term "measurement of lung volumes" usually refers to measuring the total lung capacity, residual volume, functional residual capacity, and vital capacity. These measurements are essential to the analysis of lung function and provide information that furthers the diagnostic process and the assessment of therapy. The process of measuring lung volumes can be divided into two major steps: (*a*) the determination of functional residual capacity (FRC) and (*b*) the performance of spirometry.

Determination of FRC is most commonly accomplished by using one of three basic techniques: (*a*) helium dilution, (*b*) nitrogen washout, or (*c*) body plethysmography. This chapter will discuss the fundamentals of these techniques and will also briefly discuss the use of the chest roentgenogram in measuring total lung capacity.

Forced spirometry was discussed in Chapter 1; the discussion of spirometry in this chapter will focus on the slow vital capacity and how it applies to the measurement of static lung volumes.

PHYSIOLOGY

The total lung volume can be divided into several subdivisions and compartments as shown in Figure 2.1. These subdivisions and compartments can be grouped into "volumes" and "capacities." There are four volumes: **inspiratory reserve volume (IRV), tidal volume (TV), expiratory reserve volume (ERV),** and **residual volume (RV).** Two or more of these

63

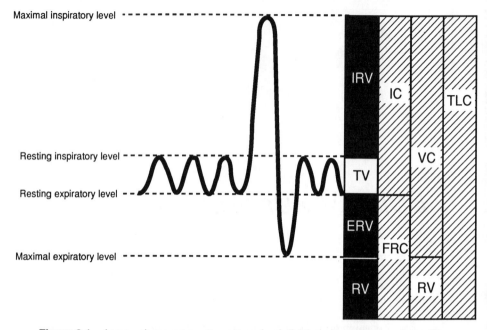

Figure 2.1. Lung volume compartments and subdivisions based on a volume-time spirogram. The four "volumes" are shaded and consist of IRV, TV, ERV, and RV. The "capacities" consist of two or more "volumes." (Modified from Forster RE, DuBois AB, Briscoe WA, Fisher AB. The lung: physiologic basis of pulmonary function tests. 3rd ed. Chicago: Year Book Medical Publishers, 1986.)

volumes make up what is called a "capacity." There are four capacities: **vital capacity (VC), inspiratory capacity (IC), functional residual capacity (FRC), and total lung capacity (TLC).**

Let me first define the four volumes. **Tidal volume** (shown in Figure 2.2*A*) is the volume of air that is inspired and expired with each breath during normal breathing. The end of the inspiratory phase is called the **end-inspiratory level**, and the end of the expiratory phase is called the **end-expiratory level.**

Inspiratory reserve volume (shown in Figure 2.2*B*) is the maximum amount of air that can be inhaled beyond the tidal volume end-inspiratory level. The **expiratory reserve volume** (shown in Figure 2.2*C*) is the maximum amount of air that can be exhaled below the tidal volume end-expiratory level.

Residual volume is the volume of air remaining in the lungs at the end of a maximum expiration. Unlike the three volumes just discussed, residual volume must be measured indirectly. First, the functional residual

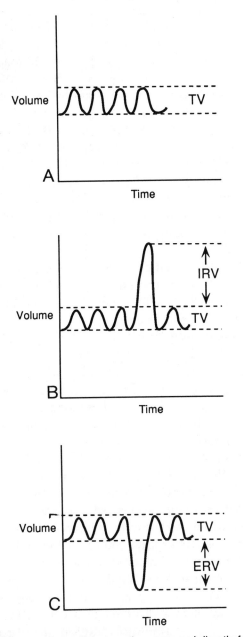

Figure 2.2. The three "volumes" that can be measured directly from the spirogram are **A**, tidal volume (TV), **B**, inspiratory reserve volume (IRV), and **C**, expiratory reserve volume (ERV).

capacity must be measured from one of several techniques. Then, from spirometry, a slow vital capacity must be obtained and divided into subdivisions (i.e., TV, IRV, ERV). Once FRC and a slow vital capacity have been performed, RV is usually calculated the following way: **RV = FRC − ERV.**

The **vital capacity** is the volume of air that can be exhaled from the lungs after a maximum inspiration. When this volume can be exhaled forcefully, it is called the **forced vital capacity (FVC)**, and when it is exhaled slowly, it is called the **slow vital capacity (SVC)**. The vital capacity can also be described as the sum of the TV, IRV, and ERV. In the healthy individual, it makes up approximately 70% of the total lung volume.

The **inspiratory capacity** is the maximum amount of air that can be inhaled from the tidal volume end-expiratory level. It is the sum of the TV and IRV. This capacity usually makes up 60 to 70% of the vital capacity in healthy individuals.

The **functional residual capacity** is the volume of air remaining in the lungs at the tidal volume end-expiratory level. As shown in Figure 2.1, the FRC consists of the ERV and RV, and its determination is a critical step in the measurement of lung volumes.

The **total lung capacity** is the volume of air in the lungs after a maximum inspiration. It consists of all four volumes—IRV, TV, ERV, and RV. It also consists of two capacities—IC and FRC.

The size of the lung volume compartments will vary depending on disease states. Thus, the measurement of these compartments helps the diagnostic process. In emphysema, for example, it is common to see a reduced FVC and FEV_1 and a reduced $FEV_1/FVC\%$ ratio. However, a patient with a restrictive process will also have a reduced FVC and FEV_1 but an increased $FEV_1/FVC\%$ ratio. Although the FEV_1/FVC ratio may be helpful in differentiating obstructive and restrictive diseases, it is not the "acid test." The only way to truly differentiate the two disease processes is to measure all the lung volume compartments. In restrictive patterns, all the compartments are reduced. In mixed (obstructive and restrictive) and obstructive disorders some compartments are reduced and some are increased. Table 2.1 shows the various compartments and their status for a particular pattern.

As noted previously, the determination of FRC is one of two main steps in determining lung volumes. The three most commonly used FRC determination techniques are (*a*) **helium dilution**, (*b*) **nitrogen washout**, and (*c*) **body plethysmography** (also called "body box"). In the healthy subject, these three methods show good agreement.[1-4] In obstructive lung disease, however, there is generally poor agreement between gas dilution techniques (helium dilution and nitrogen washout) and the body box.

Table 2.1: Lung volume compartments and their status (I-increased, D-decreased, or N-normal) for obstructive, restrictive, and mixed obstructive and restrictive lung disease patterns

	Obstructive	Restrictive	Mixed
VC	D or N	D	D
TLC	I	D	N or D
IC	N	D	N or D
FRC	I	D	N or D
ERV	D or N	D	D
RV	I	D	N or D

The gas dilution methods of helium dilution and nitrogen washout are relatively simple to perform and require little effort on the part of patients. However, these methods also have a serious weakness. In patients with obstructive lung disease, the gas dilution methods underestimate the actual FRC because they measure only those areas of the lung that are communicating with the mouth. Thus, areas that contain trapped gas are not measured. This weakness leads to a large number of obstructive lung disease patterns being falsely classified as mixed obstructive/restrictive lung disease patterns.

The body plethysmograph or body box measures the volume of gas in the thoracic cage. The body box is more expensive and technically more complicated, and it requires more cooperation and effort on the part of the patient than gas dilution methods. Nonetheless, it is also considered to be more accurate. There has been some recent evidence that the body box can overestimate FRC.[5-8] The suspected overestimation error stems from the fact that in severe obstructive lung disease, alveolar pressure is underestimated. This matter is discussed later in this chapter.

The gas dilution techniques of helium dilution and nitrogen washout are found in almost every hospital pulmonary function laboratory. The body box is used in approximately 30% of the pulmonary laboratories but is increasing in popularity because of better pricing and better computer programs, making it easier to use. The use of the chest radiograph to estimate total lung capacity has not been mentioned, but it is used in approximately 5% of the pulmonary function laboratories. It, too, is becoming increasingly popular because of improved computer hardware and software.

SPIROMETRY AND THE MEASUREMENT OF VITAL CAPACITY

The slow vital capacity is the maximum volume of air that can be slowly exhaled from the lungs after a maximum inspiration. In healthy individuals,

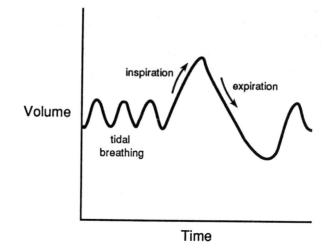

Figure 2.3. Typical slow vital capacity maneuver as expressed on a volume-time spirogram with tidal breathing followed by a maximum inspiration and then a slow complete expiration.

there is little difference between the SVC and the forced vital capacity. However, in individuals with airflow obstruction, the FVC maneuver causes gas trapping and thus is smaller than the SVC.

The instrumentation used to measure the SVC is the same instrumentation used to measured the FVC. The software of many available computerized systems has the capability to measure the SVC subdivisions.

The maneuver for performing the SVC should include several tidal breaths, followed by a maximum inspiration and then a slow complete expiration (Fig. 2.3). A variation of this maneuver ("reverse" SVC) is to again have the patient breathe several tidal breaths quietly and then reverse the steps by having the patient first slowly exhale as much air as possible from the tidal breathing level and then take a maximum inspiration (Fig. 2.4).

One additional variation in measuring the SVC is to use the concept that the vital capacity is the sum of the tidal volume, inspiratory reserve volume, and expiratory reserve volume. After breathing at tidal volume for several breaths, the patient inspires maximally and then returns to quiet breathing at tidal volume. After again breathing at tidal volume for several breaths, the patient slowly expires maximally. This "two-step" technique, as shown in Figure 2.5, measures the SVC in parts, which then can be summed.

Because the performance of the SVC, like the FVC, is effort dependent, several key points need to be reemphasized.

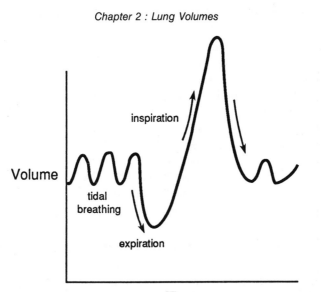

Figure 2.4. The reverse of the typical slow vital capacity is the inspiratory slow vital capacity. On a volume-time spirogram, tidal breathing is followed by a slow complete expiration and then a maximum inspiration.

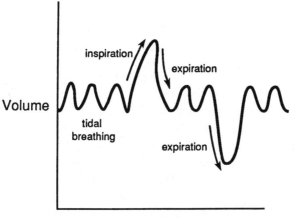

Figure 2.5. The "two-step" vital capacity, as shown on a volume-time spirogram, consists of tidal breathing followed by a maximal inspiration, then a return to tidal breathing, followed by a complete expiration.

1. Explain the purpose of the test if you have not already done so.
2. Although postponement of this test is unlikely, ensure that patient preparation and activities do not contraindicate testing. The criteria might be the same as for forced spirometry—bronchodilator inhalation, recent viral infection, serious illness, or smoking.
3. Explain the maneuver in simple terms, demonstrate, and provide feedback.

4. Use good coaching, especially near maximum inspiration and expiration levels.
5. Obtain at least two reproducible slow vital capacity maneuvers (i.e., SVC within ±5% or 100 ml, whichever is greater).
6. Obtain at least two reproducible inspiratory capacities (IC) and expiratory reserve volumes (ERV).

As mentioned previously, the vital capacity can be divided into three volumes—tidal volume, inspiratory reserve volume, and expiratory reserve volume. The ERV is commonly subtracted from the functional residual capacity to calculate residual volume. TV and IRV are commonly summed to calculate the inspiratory capacity, which is added to the FRC to calculate total lung capacity.

The reporting of slow vital capacity date is *not* standardized. One widely used method is to report the largest SVC, IC, and ERV of several trials. Another method, and the one I prefer, is to report the mean and range of several trials. Both methods, however, should report values in liters at BTPS and rounded to two decimals (e.g., 3.06 liters).

Below is an example of measurements and calculations from the SVC.

	Effort 1	Effort 2	Effort 3	Average
SVC (L)	3.20	3.33	3.29	3.27
IC (L)	2.03	2.09	2.07	2.06
TV (L)	0.60	0.64	0.61	0.62
IRV (L)	1.43	1.45	1.46	1.45
ERV (L)	1.17	1.24	1.22	1.21

It can be seen that the slow vital capacity is the sum of the three volumes (i.e., SVC = TV + IRV + ERV). Because the inspiratory capacity is the sum of tidal volume and inspiratory reserve volume (i.e., IC = TV + ERV), then the slow vital capacity is also equal to the sum of inspiratory capacity and expiratory reserve volume (i.e., SVC = IC + ERV).

The reporting of results can take the form of the largest or the average effort. If the averages are used, then the values and their ranges would be:

$$SVC = 3.27 \ (3.20–3.33)$$
$$IC \ = 2.06 \ (2.03–2.09)$$
$$ERV = 1.21 \ (1.17–1.24)$$

The advantage of expressing the mean values and the ranges is that it displays a better picture of the testing results. Still, it also takes up more room and clutters the report, and in this example the difference between the two methods of reporting is very small.

MEASUREMENT OF FRC WITH BODY PLETHYSMOGRAPHY

The **body plethysmograph** or **body box** is the first of three methods that will be discussed to measure FRC. According to Julius Comroe,[5] E. Pfluger was the first to apply Boyle's law to measure residual volume in 1882 by constructing a large metal container. The English translation of the German name for Pfluger's device was "man-box" or "man-can." However, Arthur DuBois and coworkers are usually credited with the modern-day application.[4]

In order to measure FRC by body box, the patient, sitting inside a sealed box, pants against a closed shutter. The gas volume trapped in the lungs can than be measured by applying Boyle's law. This method is generally considered to be the most accurate of the three methods because it measures the total gas volume (TGV) in the thoracic cage.

The body box is also used to measure airways resistance (Raw). The patient uses the same panting technique, or even a quiet breathing technique in some systems, but first with the shutter open and then with the shutter closed. The measurement of Raw is used to assess airflow obstruction and does not really fall under the measurement of lung volumes. Therefore, it will not be discussed.

Physiology and Instrumentation

The operating principle of the body box is based on Boyle's gas law, which states that a volume of gas at constant temperature varies inversely with the pressure applied to it:

$$P_1V_1 = P_2V_2$$

The patient sits inside the sealed body box and attaches to the mouthpiece, wears a noseclip, and breathes quietly. When a valve (shutter) to which the mouthpiece is connected is closed at the tidal volume end-expiratory position (FRC), it traps that volume of gas in the lungs. By panting in and out against the closed shutter, the patient compresses and decompresses the trapped volume while temperature remains constant. Because there is no airflow, the pressure changes and volume changes allow for the determination of the trapped volume by applying Boyle's law. The mathematics of applying Boyle's law is shown in Appendix 5.

The alveolar pressure changes caused by the compression and decompression of the lungs are estimated at the mouth. As mentioned earlier, the assumption that alveolar pressure equilibrates and is correctly measured at the mouth when the glottis is open and the cheeks are held firmly has

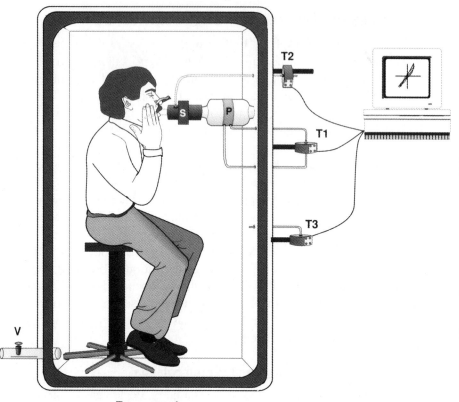

Pressure box

Figure 2.6. Pressure body plethysmograph (constant volume). The nose-clipped patient attaches to the mouthpiece and breathes through a shutter/pneumotach apparatus. The shutter (S) is open for tidal breathing and for measurements of airways resistance, and closed for measurements of thoracic gas volume. When the shutter is closed, mouth pressure is measured by a transducer (T2). The pneumotach (P) measures flow via transducer (T1), and in modern body plethysmographs the flow signal is electronically integrated to obtain volume. The body plethysmograph (or body box) pressure is measured by a transducer (T3). The signals from the three transducers are usually processed by computer. Excess body box pressure from temperature changes caused by the patient sitting in the closed "box" is vented through a valve (V).

come under recent attack.[6-9] These studies suggest that in the presence of severe airway obstruction, alveolar pressure is underestimated, resulting in an erroneously high TGV. Additionally, there has been some evidence that in patients with severe airway obstruction the panting frequency of two breaths per second may also interfere with the transmission of alveolar pressure to the mouth.[8]

This matter has not been resolved, but at the time of this writing, the accepted standard is to use the assumption that mouth pressure correctly measures alveolar pressure when the glottis is open and the cheeks are firmly held, especially in healthy individuals and patients with mild and moderate airways obstruction. The 10 to 15% overestimation of TGV in severely obstructed patients is accepted for now, but perhaps newer techniques using slower panting frequencies or even quiet breathing will become the standard in the future.

The volume changes in the body box are caused by the compression and decompression of the chest wall during the panting maneuver. The sealed box allows for the measurement of the small changes in volume (e.g., 200 to 500 ml). The three major types of body boxes, **pressure box, flow box,** and **volume box,** are classified based on how each type measures the volume change.

The **pressure box** (Fig. 2.6) uses a pressure transducer to measure body box pressure changes that are caused by the compression and decompression of the chest. It is also known as a **constant volume box**. This transducer, which is attached to the wall of the box, is calibrated by injecting known volumes into the sealed box, creating a relationship between box volume change and box pressure change. This type of box requires a correction for body weight and frequent venting of excess pressure caused by rising temperatures when the patient is inside.

The **flow box** (Fig. 2.7) measures box volume changes using a large pneumotach (which measures flow) placed in the box wall. When compression and decompression of the chest wall occur, the air in the body box will flow in and out of the penumotach. The measured flow is then integrated to get volume. The flow and mouth pressure signals must be in phase, either by mechanical adjustments or with the computer software.

The **volume box** (Fig. 2.8) measures box volume changes with an attached spirometer. It is easily calibrated by injecting a known volume into the sealed box. The frequency response of the spirometer needs to be taken into account or corrected.

In the past, the relationship between mouth pressure (which estimates alveolar pressure) and box volume changes was hand measured. Today, there is excellent software available that makes the body box an easier system to use. Additionally, software of some commercial systems also allows for the performance and measurement of slow and forced vital capacities, which provide an excellent pulmonary function testing system.

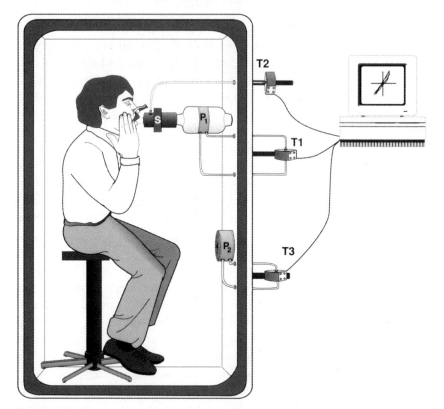

Figure 2.7. Flow body plethysmograph (variable volume). The nose-clipped patient attaches to the mouthpiece and breathes through a shutter/pneumotach apparatus. The shutter (S) is open for tidal breathing, measurement fairways resistance, and spirometry. It is closed for measurement of thoracic gas volume. When the shutter is closed, mouth pressure is measured by a transducer (T2). The pneumotach (P1) measures flow via transducer T1. Flow can then be electronically integrated to obtain volume. Modem computer programs allow the user to perform slow and forced vital capacities. Changes in plethysmograph (body box) volume, which occur with chest-wall movement, are measured by electronic integration of flow through pneumotach P2 and transducer T3. The signals from the three transducers are usually processed by computer.

Technique

The body box should be calibrated every day it is used. The opera-tor's manual should describe the calibration process, and it should be followed. Usually the process consists of calibrating the three transducer-amplifier circuits; mouth pressure, box volume, and flow. The computer-ization of this process has greatly simplified and improved the calibration

Volume box

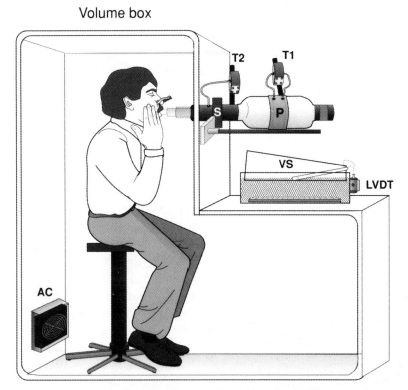

Figure 2.8. Volume body plethysmograph (variable volume). The nose-clipped patient attaches to the mouthpiece and breathes through a shutter/pneumotach apparatus, which is usually located outside the plethysmograph (body box). The shutter (S) is open for tidal breathing, measurement of airway resistance, and spirometry. It is closed for measurement of thoracic gas volume. When the shutter is closed, mouth pressure is measured by a transducer (T2). The pneumotach (P) measures flow via transducer T1. Flow can then be electronically integrated to obtain volume. Changes in body box volume, which occur with chest-wall movement, are measured by a volume-displacement spirometer (VS) and a linear volume-displacement transducer (LVDT). The type of spirometer shown is a Krogh water-sealed spirometer. Signal processing is usually done by computer, and modern programs allow the user to perform slow and forced vital capacities.

procedure. A log of calibration results should be maintained, showing date, calibration values, barometric pressure, and technician initials.

Patient preparation for measuring FRC in the body box begins with some instructions before he/she enters the box. These should include how the patient should use the mouthpiece and noseclips and the fact that the patient will sit inside and that the door will be closed. Many patients are apprehensive about being "closed in" in a small space. The technician should assure the individual that the door can be opened at any time between maneuvers. Additionally, most boxes available today are constructed partly with clear plexiglass, which offers a feeling of openness.

The panting maneuver must also be explained. Usually the patient is asked to pant (shallow breaths) at a rate of one to two breaths per second. When the shutter closes and airflow stops, panting is more difficult. The technician should explain that although air movement really stops when the shutter closes, it is the pressure of the panting that is being measured and therefore the patient must continue the panting maneuver. The technician should then demonstrate with his/her own mouth and lips the open (if Raw is to be measured) and closed shutter maneuvers.

Practicing with the patient is the next step. With the door closed and sealed, communication is hampered. Most of the intercom systems on the boxes do not provide good sound quality and, therefore, can cause delays as the patient tries to understand and perform this tricky maneuver. My recommendation is to leave the door open and show the patient what it feels like to pant against the closed shutter, as well as giving the patient additional instructions or suggestions. Once it is thought that the patient is ready, the technician should seal the door and proceed with the testing. The patient still may have some problems (described below) with the maneuver, but any "fine-tuning" can be done over the intercom system.

The common problems encountered in getting the patient to do the panting maneuver correctly include incorrect panting frequency (i.e., too fast or too slow), failure to inspire and expire against the closed shutter, panting too hard, lips failing to seal around the mouthpiece, and glottis closure. Additionally, unsatisfactory results may occur when the patient allows his/her cheeks to "puff in and out" with the closed shutter panting. This is corrected by having the patient place his/her own hands on the cheeks and hold them from moving as shown in Figure 2.9.

The desired measurement is thoracic gas volume at functional residual capacity (TGV at FRC). This is accomplished by having the patient breathe quietly for several breaths and then closing the shutter at precisely tidal volume end-expiratory level and instructing the patient to pant. In most commercial systems the closing of the shutter is handled by the computer, reducing timing errors.

The body boxes available today have some very sophisticated and creative software. Usually, the mouth pressure/box volume relationship is displayed for inspection, and the computer estimate of the slope of this relationship can be accepted or modified by the technician. The calculation of TGV at FRC is automatically done. If spirometry can be performed with the

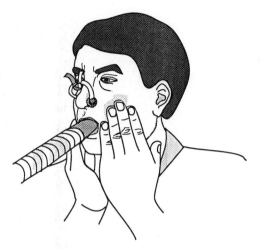

Figure 2.9. To keep a patient's cheeks from "puffing in and out" during the closed shutter maneuver, his/her hands should be placed on the cheeks and pressed firmly toward the face.

available software, usually all the lung volume compartments are also displayed.

The technician should acquire at least five estimates of TGV at FRC. The author's recommendation for acceptable agreement among the TGV determinations is to be within ±10% of the mean value. The mean TGV should be reported. As stated earlier, the method for determining which SVC and other lung volumes to report is controversial. For example with total lung capacity, the highest or mean value of several efforts could be placed on the final or summary report. For residual volume, on the other hand, the lowest, highest, or mean value of several measurements could be used. The author recommends reporting mean values of the lung volume compartments (TLC, IC, FRC, ERV, RV, SVC) with the range of values obtained if space permits.

MEASUREMENT OF FRC BY HELIUM DILUTION

A second method for determining FRC is by **closed-circuit helium dilution.**[10] This method involves diluting an inert gas, such as helium or neon, in the lungs. This dilution process is accomplished by rebreathing the gas in a closed system over a short period of time (usually 2 to 10 minutes).

This method is widely used in pulmonary function laboratories for several reasons. It is a very easy test for the patient, since it requires only tidal breathing and minimal learning and effort. The instrumentation is simple and inexpensive, requiring only a gas analyzer and spirometer. As mentioned earlier, the major drawback of this method is that unlike the body box method, it measures only the lung volume that is in communication with the mouth. This becomes a problem in patients with airflow obstruction and results in an underestimation of FRC, which leads to an underestimation of RV and TLC.

Physiology and Instrumentation

The closed-circuit helium dilution technique uses a spirometer and breathing circuit that contains a known volume (V_s) and concentration (C_s) of helium (Fig. 2.10). The patient, wearing noseclips, is connected to the mouthpiece. After a valve is opened (connecting the patient to the spirometer and helium), the patient breathes into and out of this closed spirometer circuit. If the patient is "turned in" to the spirometer and helium at tidal volume end-expiratory level (FRC), then the volume in the lung (V_L) that will be measured is FRC. However, the patient could be "turned in" above or below FRC, allowing for the measurement of a lung volume other than FRC.

It is critical, in this closed circuit, that the circuit volume at the start of the test equal the circuit volume at the end of the test. Therefore, the patient's exhaled carbon dioxide (CO_2) must be absorbed, and oxygen (O_2) must be added in amounts that equal the patient's oxygen consumption.

The rebreathing continues until the helium concentration is equilibrated as shown in Figure 2.10. In healthy patients, equilibration time takes approximately 2 to 3 minutes. However, in patients with obstructive lung disease, the equilibration time can take 5 to 10 minutes. One technique that is sometimes used to speed up the testing time is a periodic deep breath. Equilibration is usually defined by a plateau in the helium concentration (no change for 60 seconds).

The initial concentration of helium in the spirometer (C_s) is diluted proportionately by the addition of the patient's lung volume (V_L), resulting in a final helium concentration that reflects the concentration in both the spirometer circuit and the lungs (C_{LS}). Looking at this mathematically, it can be seen that:

$$\text{Volumes and concentrations at beginning of test} = \text{Volumes and concentrations at end of test}$$

$$V_s C_s + V_L C_L = V_s C_{LS} + V_L C_{LS}$$

Because $C_L = 0$ at the beginning of test

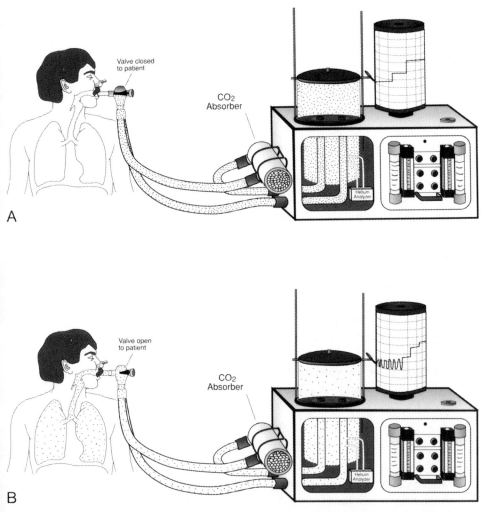

Figure 2.10. Closed-circuit helium dilution for determination of functional residual capacity. **A**, The known concentration and volume of helium in the spirometer system is separated from the patient by a closed valve. **B**, The valve is opened and helium (indicated with dots) is redistributed by rebreathing until it is equilibrated in lungs and circuit.

$$V_S C_L = V_S C_{LS} + V_L C_{LS}$$

Solving for V_L

$$V_L = \frac{V_S C_{LS} - C_{LS} V_S}{C_{LS}}$$

$$V_L = \frac{V_s(C_s - C_{LS})}{C_{LS}}$$

or, simplified

$$FRC = \frac{V_s(C_1 - C_2)}{C_2} - He\ Abs.\ Corr.$$

Where V_s = volume in spirometer and circuit; V_L = volume in lung; C_s = concentration of helium in spirometer, also called C_1; C_L = concentration of helium in lung; C_{LS} = concentration of helium after equilibration of lungs and spirometer, also called C_2; He Abs. Corr. = volume of helium absorption by the blood during rebreathing (usually 0.1 liter).

The volume in the spirometer and circuit (V_s) includes the known volume of helium and a "dead space" that consists of the tubing, the analyzer, and the space in the CO_2 absorber. This "dead space" must be measured.

In most automated systems, this is accomplished by initially adding a small amount of helium to the closed circuit and taking an initial reading. A known volume of air is then added, and after a short time to allow equilibration, a second helium concentration reading is taken. Using the dilution equation above, the V_s can be calculated. The patient is then connected and "turned in" to the closed-circuit system, and, after equilibration, a third helium concentration reading is taken. When this three-reading process is combined into one equation, it becomes:

$$FRC = \frac{C_1}{C_2} \times \frac{C_2 - C_3}{C_1 - C_2} \times V_{ADDED} - He\ Abs.\ Corr.$$

Where C_1 = concentration of helium in spirometer and circuit; C_2 = concentration of helium in spirometer and circuit after a known volume of air is added; C_3 = concentration of helium in spirometer and circuit after equilibration of lungs and spirometer system; V_{ADDED} = volume of air added to spirometer and circuit between C_1 and C_2; He Abs. Corr. = volume of helium absorbed by the blood during rebreathing (usually 0.1 liter).

An example of calculating an FRC by closed-circuit helium dilution is shown below:

Volume of air added	= 1.20 liters
Initial helium concentration (C_1)	= 10.0%
Helium concentration after air added (C_2)	= 8.6%
Helium concentration after patient equilibration (C_3)	= 6.2%
Spirometer temperature	= 23°C

Helium absorbtion correction = 0.1 liter

Switching error = 0

$$FRC = \frac{C_1}{C_2} \times \frac{C_2 - C_3}{C_1 - C_2} \times V_{ADDED} - He\ Abs.\ Corr.$$

$$FRC = \frac{10.0}{8.6} \times \frac{8.6 - 6.2}{10.0 - 8.6} \times 1.20_{ATPS} - 0.10$$

$$FRC = 1.16 \times \frac{2.4}{1.4} \times 1.20 - 0.10$$

$$FRC = 2.28 \times BTPS\ factor$$

$$FRC = 2.47\ liters$$

The **helium analyzer** used in these systems operates on a thermal conductivity principle. This principle is based on the fact that gases are able to conduct heat. Different gases conduct at different rates. By introducing gas molecules into a sampling chamber containing a heated wire, the temperature of that wire decreases, allowing more current to flow through the wire. In order to be specific for helium, other gases must either be removed or be compared to a reference. Therefore, CO_2 and water are "scrubbed" from the sample gas, and oxygen and nitrogen are negated by comparing the thermal conductivity of the sample gas to a dry room-air reference. A Wheatstone bridge is incorporated to measure the resistance difference of the sample and reference chambers.

Technique

The spirometer used for helium dilution systems should be calibrated as recommended by the manufacturer and leak tested every day it is used. The CO_2 and water absorbers should be fresh.

Patients should be seated comfortably and told how to use the mouthpiece and noseclips. They should be told that the test requires sitting quietly and breathing through the mouthpiece with lips tightly sealed for several minutes. They should be reminded not to remove the mouthpiece until told to do so. The technician should also mention that periodic deep breaths may be needed.

With patients nose-clipped and breathing room air while attached to the mouthpiece, observe their tidal breathing for several breaths. If unable to see chest movement, the technician can place a hand on the patient's back or shoulder to feel the movement. Turn the valve that connects the patients to the spirometer system at tidal volume end-expiratory level (FRC). If the valve is not turned at exactly FRC, a "switching error" correction will be necessary.

The CO_2 produced by the patient is continually being absorbed as the helium mixture circulates in the spirometer, circuit, and patient. Oxygen is added by one of two techniques. The first is a **continuous-addition technique**, which keeps the spirometer system volume constant by continually adding oxygen in small quantities that equal the volume loss caused by the patient's O_2 consumption. Typically, an adult patient on these systems has an O_2 consumption of 300 to 600 ml/min.

The second oxygen addition technique is the **bulk-addition technique**. Systems that use this technique put a bolus of oxygen (e.g., 1000 ml) into the spirometer before the patient is turned in. Once the patient is turned in, all of the added oxygen must be consumed before the test can be ended. Otherwise the volume of the spirometer and circuit will have changed, causing a greater helium concentration change than would normally be seen.

Of the two techniques for O_2 addition, the bulk-addition technique is easier because it is done once and the technician need only remember to end the test after all the O_2 has been consumed. The drawback is that if equilibration has not been achieved (i.e., the helium concentration has not plateaued) and all of the O_2 bolus has been consumed, another bolus will have to be added and patients must then be allowed to continue to rebreathe until the second bolus has been consumed. The continuous-addition technique has been greatly simplified on the new instruments because of computerization and probably is the preferred method among users.

The technician should perform at least two helium dilution determinations of FRC separated by 5 to 10 minutes. The author's recommendation for acceptable agreement is ±10%. The mean FRC should be reported in liters at BTPS, rounded to two decimals (e.g., 3.13 liters).

MEASUREMENT OF FRC BY NITROGEN WASHOUT

The third method of determining FRC is the open-circuit nitrogen washout. This method involves removing or "washing out" the nitrogen (N_2) gas present in a patient's lungs. This is done by having the patient breathe 100% oxygen for several minutes. Like the helium dilution method, this method is widely used in pulmonary function laboratories. It is easy for the patient to perform and requires minimal learning and effort. Also like the helium dilution method, the N_2 washout method has the drawback of only measuring the lung spaces that communicate with the mouth. Thus it too underestimates FRC in patients with airflow obstruction.

Physiology and Instrumentation

The early modern technique[11] for the open-circuit method used the apparatus shown in Figure 2.11. This technique, cumbersome compared to today's techniques, had the patient breathe while attached to a mouthpiece and exhale maximally, at which time an alveolar gas sample was taken that represented an attempt to measure the average lung N_2 concentration on room air. Following this sample, the patient breathed room air for two more minutes to restore quiet breathing. Then, a valve was turned at FRC so that the patient could breathe 100% oxygen from a reservoir bag for 7 minutes. The exhaled gas was collected in a 100-liter gasometer (Tissot). At the conclusion of 7 minutes, the patient was instructed to exhale fully and another alveolar sample was taken. The patient was then disconnected, the breathing circuit was flushed, and a gas sample was taken from the gasometer.

The three N_2 samples were analyzed using the volumetric methods (e.g., Van Slyke manometer), which depended on chemical absorption. This process, which was commonplace in the early 1960s, took 10 to 20 minutes for each sample and was extremely technique dependent.

Today, the large gasometer has been replaced by flow meters, and the volumetric gas analyzers have been replaced by electronic nitrogen analyzers that can analyze the N_2 concentration of each breath. Additionally, the second alveolar sample at the end of the oxygen-breathing period has been eliminated from the technique.

The concept of the N_2 washout is based on the fact that at the start of the test the unknown FRC that is being determined contains 80% N_2 and an unknown concentration of O_2 (probably between 16 and 21%) and CO_2 (probably between 0.4 and 5.0%). By measuring the volume of N_2 in the FRC and applying a concentration dilution formula, the FRC volume can be determined. Thus,

$$C_1V_1 \; = \; C_2V_2$$

Where C_1 = N_2 concentration in the FRC at start of test; V_1 = FRC volume; C_2 = N_2 concentration in exhaled volume; V_2 = total exhaled volume during oxygen-breathing period.

As stated earlier, the N_2 washout measures the lung volume that can be ventilated by the mouth. Thus, those patients with large amounts of trapped

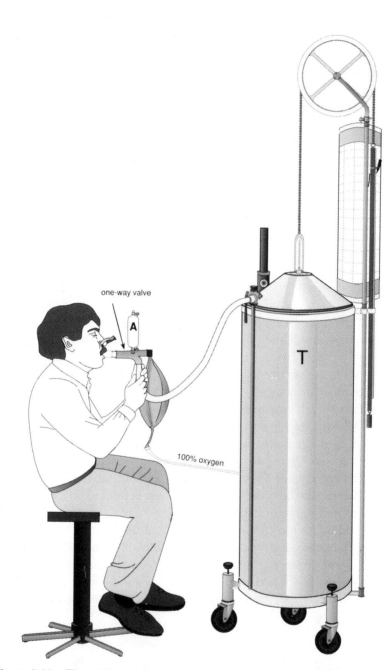

Figure 2.11. The early modern open-circuit nitrogen washout circuit for determination of functional residual capacity. The patient breathes through a one-way valve, to which is connected a vacuum bottle (A) for collecting the alveolar sample. The inspiratory side is connected to a 100% oxygen reservoir, and the expiratory side is connected to a large water-sealed spirometer (T). This spirometer, which is also known as a "Tissot" (pronounced tee-so), is usually 100 to 200 liters—enough capability to collect the expired air during 7 minutes of quiet breathing.

air or areas of lung that are poorly ventilated will have an underestimated FRC. It was shown in the early papers[11,12] that increased breathing periods (11 to 15 minutes) obtained larger FRCs in patients with obstructive lung disease. However, the use of longer periods of time is more uncomfortable for the patient, and there is a concern that in some patients breathing 100% oxygen for more than a few minutes may depress the ventilatory drive.

The nitrogen analyzer that is used with modern systems operates on a photoelectric principle. Gas is pulled through a needle valve into an ionization chamber by a vacuum pump. The molecules are ionized and emit a light. This light is then filtered and collected by a photoresistor, which converts the light into an electrical signal. The intensity of the light is directly related to the concentration of N_2 in the sample.

The use of the computer has allowed for the signal from the N_2 analyzer to be combined with the volume signal from a spirometer to provide instantaneous or breath-by-breath measurements of N_2 volume. This technology allows for faster detection of leaks, which is an advantage over the helium dilution technique.

The computerization of this technique has also shortened the time required for calculation of FRC. The basic equation used with the early technique was:

$$FRC = \left(\frac{(\text{Tissot volume})(FEN_2 - FIN_2)}{FAN_{2initial} - FAN_{2final}} \right) - DS$$

An example of calculating an FRC by nitrogen washout using the above equation is shown below. An open-circuit N_2 washout was performed with the patient inspiring 100% O_2 and the exhaled air collected in a 120-liter Tissot gasometer. The following information was obtained:

Barometric pressure	= 631 mm Hg
Tissot temperature (T)	= 24°C
Tissot volume after 7 minutes of breathing	= 56.3 liters ATPS
FEN_2 (fractional concentration of expired N_2 in Tissot)	= 0.0368
FIN_2 (fractional concentration of inspired N_2)	= 0.001
$FAN_{2initial}$ (alveolar N_2 concentration at start of test)	= 0.80
FAN_{2final} (alveolar N_2 concentration at end of test)	= 0.015
DS (valve dead space, liters)	= 0.090

$$FRC = \frac{(\text{Tissot volume})(FEN_2 - FIN_2)}{FAN_{2initial} - FAN_{2final}} - DS$$

VE_{Tissot} (i.e., Tissot volume at ATPS including system dead space)

= 56.3 liters

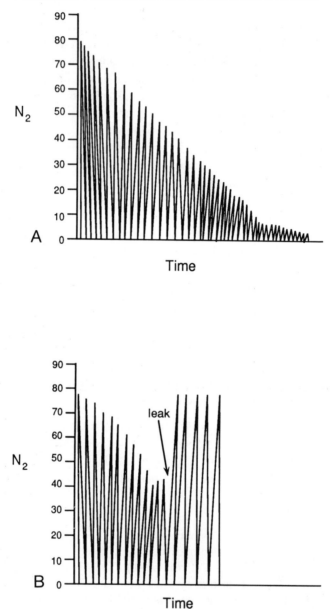

Figure 2.12. **A,** A typical tracing of a nitrogen washout test using nitrogen analyzer. **B,** When leaks occur (e.g., the patient does not keep his/her lips sealed tightly) room air enters the circuit and the concentration of nitrogen returns to approximately 78%.

$$VE_{Tissot} \text{ at BTPS} = VE_{Tissot} \text{ at ATPS} \times \frac{310}{273 + T} \times \frac{PB - PH_2O \text{ at } 24°C}{PB - PH_2O \text{ at } 37°C}$$

$$VE_{Tissot} \text{ at BTPS} = 56.3 \times \frac{310}{273 + 24} \times \frac{631 - 22}{631 - 47}$$

$$VE_{Tissot} \text{ at BTPS} = 56.3 \times 1.044 \times 1.043$$

$$VE_{Tissot} \text{ at BTPS} = 61.30 \text{ liters}$$

$$FRC = \frac{(61.30)(0.0368 - 0.001)}{0.80 - 0.015}$$

$$FRC = \frac{(61.30)(0.0358)}{0.785} = 2.80 \text{ liters at BTPS}$$

Technique

The flow-meter device and N_2 analyzer should always be calibrated every day of use. Patients should be seated comfortably and given instructions on how to use the mouthpiece and noseclips. They should be told that the test requires sitting quietly and breathing on the mouthpiece with lips tightly sealed for several minutes. They should be reminded to keep the mouthpiece in place with lips sealed until told by the technician to remove it.

Patients should then be observed for several breaths prior to "turn in." This is to insure that the "turn in" to the 100% O_2 occurs at tidal volume end-expiration level (FRC). The test is usually ended when the expired N_2 concentration falls below a certain level. This level is between 1.0 and 1.5%, and one recommendation is 1.2%.[13]

The N_2 concentration should be monitored throughout the test. When no leaks are present, the N_2 concentration would appear as shown in Figure 2.12A. If a leak occurs, N_2 from room air enters the system, and the N_2 concentration abruptly rises as shown in Figure 2.12B.

The N_2 washout procedure should be repeated with a 10-minute interval between trials until two FRC measurements that agree within 10% are obtained. The mean FRC of the measurements that agree within 10% should be reported in liters at BTPS, rounded to two decimals (e.g., 3.78 liters).

DETERMINATION OF LUNG VOLUMES BY ROENTGENOGRAM

Two basic methods have been described to use the chest roentgenogram (radiograph) to measure lung volumes: (a) the planimeter method[14,15] and (b) the ellipse method.[16]

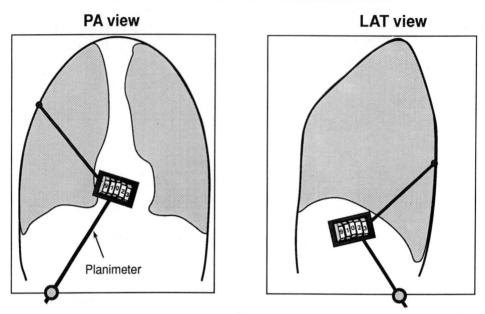

Figure 2.13. Measurement of total lung capacity from chest roentgenogram using the planimetry technique. The two-armed planimeter is placed on the PA and LAT view of the chest at full inspiration. With one end fixed, the other end is used to trace the periphery of each view. A mechanical counter measures the distance traveled, which can be converted to volume.

A planimeter is a device with two arms that pivot around a fixed point allowing one to trace over the lines of any two-dimensional shape (Fig. 2.13). By outlining all the lung fields in the posteroanterior (PA) and lateral (LAT) films including the heart but excluding the sternum, the roentgenographic chest volume can be calculated.

The ellipse method assumes that the lungs can be divided into a large number of elliptical cross sections (Fig. 2.14). The area of the elliptical sections is determined from the PA and LAT view chest films and then converted to volume. The area of the heart, the domes of the diaphragm, and the pulmonary blood and tissue are subtracted out.

Both methods have compared well to each other as well as to TLC measured by plethysmographic and dilution techniques.[17-20]

The drawbacks of using the chest film are (*a*) only TLC can be measured, and (*b*) TLC can be underestimated if the patient does not maximally inspire when the film is taken. Additionally, the technique is dependent on a good quality film in order to define the lung boundaries.

PA view   **LAT view**

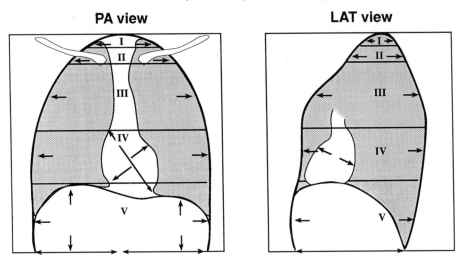

Figure 2.14. Measurement of total lung capacity from chest roentgenograms using the ellipse method. The PA and LAT views of the chest at full inspiration are divided into five elliptical cross sections or segments. The area of each section is measured (arrows indicate the points between which to measure) and then converted to volume.

However, the advantages of being unaffected by poorly ventilated areas and the ability to retrospectively compare films when pulmonary function tests are not available or comparable make this technique valuable. The use of computers has shortened the time required to measure and calculate, and, in all likelihood, the computer will make this technique more popular in the future.

REFERENCE VALUES

As in forced spirometry, it is common practice to report reference or predicted values for static lung volumes. A recent survey[21] found that the most commonly used study for lung volume reference values was that of Goldman and Becklake.[22] This study used hydrogen dilution (similar to helium dilution) to measure FRC on 44 male and 50 female subjects near Johannesburg, South Africa (altitude 5700 feet). The reference equations from that and other studies are listed in Appendix 4.

The techniques used in the many reference studies vary and include helium dilution, hydrogen dilution, nitrogen washout, single breath helium dilution, and body plethysmography.[22-26] The criteria for choosing a particular reference equation for one's laboratory should include similar equipment and methods and similar populations. Once a choice has been made,

Table 2.2: Office pulmonary function data before and after bronchodilator

	Before		After
TLC (L)	4.63	(96)*	
FRC (L)**	2.58	(92)	
RV (L)	2.08	(109)	
SVC (L)	2.55	(71)	
FVC (L)	2.18	(60)	2.38
FEV₁ (L)	1.08	(42)	1.18
FEV₁/FVC (%)	50		50
FEF 25-75% (L/S)	0.65	(26)	0.67

* Values in parentheses are percent of predicted.
** Measured by helium dilution.

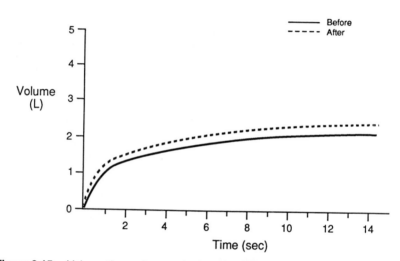
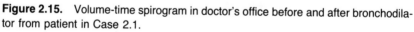

Figure 2.15. Volume-time spirogram in doctor's office before and after bronchodilator from patient in Case 2.1.

a laboratory should consider comparing 10 to 20 healthy subjects selected from its population with the reference values. If the differences between the 10 to 20 healthy subjects and reference values are small (e.g., ±10%), then the laboratory can be reasonably confident that the chosen reference values are appropriate.

CASE 2.1

A 68-year-old white female with a complaint of worsening dyspnea was seen in the pulmonologist's office. She admitted to having been a heavy smoker (90 pack-years—a pack-year is one package of cigarettes per day for 1 year) but

Table 2.3: Hospital pulmonary function data before and after bronchodilator

	Before		After
TLC (L)	5.76	(120)*	
FRC (L) **	3.97	(142)	
RV (L)	3.13	(164)	
SVC (L)	2.63	(73)	2.68
FVC (L)	2.28	(63)	2.43
FEV₁ (L)	1.11	(43)	1.29
FEV₁/FVC (%)	49		53
FEF25-75% (L/S)	0.59	(24)	0.83
Raw (cm H₂O/L/S)	2.93		1.84
SGaw (L/cm H₂O/L/S)	0.07		0.13
DLCO	17.30	(74)	
DLCO/VA	3.64	(75)	

* Values in parentheses are percent of predicted.
** Measured body plethysmograph.

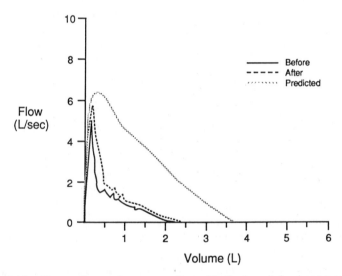

Figure 2.16.　Flow-volume spirogram performed in the hospital pulmonary function laboratory showing before and after bronchodilator, as well as the predicted curve from patient in Case 2.1.

had recently quit. This office was equipped to measure spirometry and lung volumes, and the results of her tests are shown in Table 2.2, and Figure 2.15. Her chest film had an emphysematous appearance with increased diameters. After seeing the results of the office pulmonary function test, the doctor ordered another test at the area hospital, and the results are shown in Table 2.3, and Figure 2.16.

Questions

1. How would you interpret the pulmonary function tests done in the doctor's office?
2. How would you interpret the pulmonary function tests done in the hospital, and why does the interpretation change?

Answers and Discussion

1. The pulmonary function test data done in the office and shown in Table 2.3 reveal normal lung volumes (TLC, FRC, and RV) and a reduced SVC. The data also reveal severe airflow limitation with a minimal response to bronchodilator. There is a question as to why the lung volumes do not reveal hyperinflation that would be consistent with this degree of obstruction and the chest film interpretation. Therefore, the final interpretation would most likely state a mixed obstructive and restrictive disorder.

2. The pulmonary function test data from the hospital use the body plethysmograph and show a different picture. There is still severe airflow limitation and the diffusing capacity is reduced, but the lung volumes are all markedly increased. There is a good response to bronchodilator. The final interpretation from this data is that of severe airflow limitation but certainly not a mixed disorder.

The major difference between the two interpretations is dependent on the measurement of FRC. In the doctor's office, the FRC (2.55 liters) was measured by helium dilution. In the hospital laboratory, the FRC (3.97 liters) is significantly higher.

Why are the two FRC determinations so different? The helium dilution method is a gas dilution technique that is commonly used in the determination of FRC. It requires that the patient breathe into a system that contains a known volume and concentration of helium. During the breathing period, the helium diffuses and equilibrates into the gas spaces of the lung that communicate with the mouth. Noncommunicating spaces are not measured. Thus, the FRC can be underestimated.

The body plethysmograph (body box) is another method to determine FRC. Although expensive and requiring more technical expertise, it is quick and accurate. It measures the total gas volume in the thoracic cage at the time a shutter is closed. This volume includes noncommunicating areas and therefore is more accurate than the gas dilution technique.

The difference between the two sets of lung volumes in this patient can be accounted for by the presence of trapped gas spaces or poorly communicating airways. The correct interpretation is that the patient is hyperinflated and does not have a mixed disorder.

CASE 2.2

A 58-year-old black male office worker was tested in the pulmonary function laboratory. Spirometry at a recent physical exam in the doctor's office detected

Table 2.4: Pulmonary function values before and after bronchodilator in the pulmonary function laboratory

	Before		After
FVC (L)	3.78	(75)*	3.93
FEV₁ (L)	2.00	(57)	2.12
FEV₁/FVC (%)	53		54
FEF25-75% (L/S)	2.34	(59)	2.79
FRC$_{body\ plethysmograph}$ (L)	2.89	(72)	
RV (L)	1.94	(103)	
TLC (L)	5.85	(85)	
SVC (L)	3.91	(78)	
Raw (cm H₂O/L/S)	2.13		1.92
Gaw/TGV	0.15		0.19

* Values in parentheses are percent of predicted.

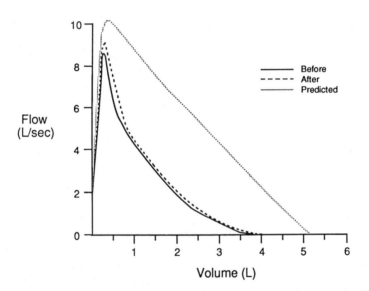

Figure 2.17. Flow-volume spirogram showing before and after bronchodilator curves as well as the reference (i.e., predicted) curve.

some "abnormal" results. He denied shortness of breath or cough but claimed to be a 40 pack-year smoker. His laboratory results are shown in Table 2.4 and Figure 2.17.

Questions:
1. What is the interpretation/evaluation of these pulmonary function tests?
2. What issues should be raised with the reference values?

Table 2.5: Pulmonary function values before and after bronchodilator

	Before		After
FVC (L)	3.78	(95)*	3.93
FEV$_1$ (L)	2.00	(71)	2.12
FEV$_1$/FVC (%)	53		54
FEF25-75% (L/S)	2.34	(65)	2.79
FRC$_{body\ plethysmograph}$ (L)	2.89	(88)	
RV (L)	1.94	(95)	
TLC (L)	5.85	(97)	
SVC (L)	3.91	(98)	
Raw (cm H$_2$O/L/S)	2.13		1.92
Gaw/TGV	0.15		0.19

* Values in parenthesis are percent of predicted.

Answers and Discussion:

The data from Table 2.4 and Figure 2.17 reveal airflow limitation, without a meaningful response to bronchodilator. Additionally, the lung volumes are reduced, suggesting a mixed obstructive and restrictive disorder.

The predicted or reference values used by the laboratory do not state whether they are race specific. If they are based on a Caucasian population, then the apparent restrictive process could be an "artifact."

Healthy or "normal" values for pulmonary function tests are frequently based on entirely Caucasian populations. The predicted values for the lung volumes (TLC, RV, FRC) shown in Table 2.4 come from a study by Goldman and Becklake,[22] and the other predicted values come from a study by Morris.[27] Neither of these particular studies states the race or ethnic background of the subjects who participated.

There have been several studies that have documented that blacks have lower lung volumes than whites.[28-32] This has been attributed to the fact that blacks have longer legs and shorter trunks. Thus, standing height, which is a major factor in predicting pulmonary function values, is biased.

When the predicted values are recalculated (shown in Table 2.5) based on the studies of Rossiter[30] and Stinson,[31] which used black populations, the interpretation changes to airflow limitation.

In practice, most pulmonary function laboratories use scaling factors when testing blacks. The usual process adjusts the Caucasian population predicted values down approximately 15%. This approach has a major pitfall, in that the 15% correction is an average. The difference between Caucasian and black values varies with each parameter. For TLCs, for example, blacks have approximately 11% lower predicted values.[30]

A pulmonary function laboratory must give careful consideration to the selection of predicted values. The use of race-specific predicted equations raises the issue of whether the available studies are adequate, because they do not provide criteria for determining race. In many studies, the assumption is made that racial identity is evident through "color" distinctions. However, this may not always be true in practice.

The alternative to race-specific predicted values is to take racial issues into of the date in Table 2.5 might have read "airflow limitation without meaningful response to bronchodilators and normal lung volumes when corrected for race."

The important consideration is that there is a weakness of using healthy reference equations based on Caucasian populations for non-Caucasian patients. If race-specific reference equations are used, it should be noted on report.

REFERENCES

1. Tierney DF, Nadel JA. Concurrent measurements of functional residual capacity by three methods. J Appl Physiol 1962; 17:871–873.

2. Reichel G. Differences between intrathoracic gas measured by the body plethysmograph and functional residual capacity determined by gas dilution methods. Prog Respir Res 1968;4:188–193.

3. Cobeel LJ. Comparison between measurement of functional residual capacity and thoracic gas volume in chronic obstructive pulmonary disease. Prog Respir Res 1969;4:194–204.

4. DuBois AB, Botelho SV, Bedel GN, et al. A rapid plethysmographic method for measuring thoracic gas volume: a comparison with a nitrogen washout method for measuring FRC in normal subjects. J Clin Invest 1956;35:322–326.

5. Comroe J. Retrospectroscope. Man-Cans. Am Rev Respir Dis 1977;116:945–950.

6. Rodenstein DO, Stanescu DC. Reassessment of lung volume measurement by helium dilution and body plethysmography in chronic airflow obstruction. Am Rev Respir Dis 1982;126:1040–1044.

7. Rodenstein DO, Stanescu DC, Francis C. Demonstration of failure of body plethysmography in airway obstruction. J Appl Physiol 1982;52:949–954.

8. Shore SA, Huk O, Mannix S, Martin JG. Effect of panting frequency on the plethysmographic determination of thoracic gas volume in chronic obstructive pulmonary disease. Am Rev Respir Dis 1983;128:54–59.

9. Shore S, Milic-Emili J, Martin JG. Reassessment of body plethysmographic techique for the measurement of thoracic gas volume in asthmatics. Am Rev Respir Dis 1982;126:515–520.

10. Meneely GR, Ball COT, Kory RC, et al. A simplified closed circuit helium dilution method for the determination of the residual volume of the lungs. Am J Med 1960;28:824–831.

11. Darling RC, Cournand A. Richards DW Jr. Studies on the intrapulmonary mixture of gases. III. An open circuit method for measuring residual air. J. Clin Invest 1940;19:609–618.

12. Emmanuel G, Briscoe A, Cournand A. A method for the determination of the volume of air in the lungs: measurements in chronic pulmonary emphysema. J Clin Invest 1961;20:329–337.

13. Clausen J, ed. Pulmonary function testing: guidelines and controversies. New York: Academic Press, 1982:115–127.

14. Hurtado A, Fray WN. Studies of total pulmonary capacity and its subdivisions. II. Correlation with physical and radiologic measurements. J Clin Invest 1933; 12:807–823.

15. Pratt PC, Klugh GA. A method for the determination of total lung capacity from posteroanterior and lateral chest

roentgenograms. Am Rev Respir Dis 1967;96:548–552.

16. Barnhard HJ, Pierce JA, Joyce JW, Bates JH. Roentgenographic determination of total lung capacity. Am J Med 1960;28: 51–60.

17. Harris TR, Pratt PC, Kilburn KH. Total lung capacity measured by roentgenograms. Am J Med 1971;50:756–763.

18. Ries AL, Clausen JL, Friedman PJ. Measurement of lung volumes from supine portable chest radiographs. J Appl Physiol 1979;47:1332–1335.

19. Pierce RJ, Brown DJ, Holmes M, Cumming G, Denison DM. Estimation of lung volumes from chest radiographs using shape formation. Thorax 1979;34: 726–734.

20. Miller RD, Offord KP. Roentgenologic determination of total lung capacity. Mayo Clin Proc 1980;55:694–699.

21. Ghio AJ, Crapo RO, Elliott CG. Reference equations used to predict pulmonary function. Chest 1990;97:400–403.

22. Goldman HI, Becklake MR. Respiratory function tests: normal values at median altitudes and the prediction of normal results. Am Rev Tubercul 1959;79:457–467.

23. Grimby G. Soderholm B. Spirometric studies in normal subjects. III. Static lung volumes and maximum voluntary ventilation in adults with a note on physical fitness. Acta Medica Scand 1963;173:199–206.

24. Boren HG, Kory RC, Syner JC. The veterans administrative-army cooperative study of pulmonary function. II. The lung volume and its subdivisions in normal men. Am J Med 1966;41:96–114.

25. Crapo RO, Morris AH, Clayton PD, Nixon CR. Lung volumes in healthy nonsmoking adults. Bull Eur Physiopathol Respir 1982;18:419–425.

26. Viljanen A, ed. Reference values for body plethysmography in non-smoking, healthy adults. Scand J Clin Lab Invest 1982;42(suppl):35–50.

27. Morris JF, Koski A, Johnson LC. Spirometric standards for healthy nonsmoking adults. Am Rev Respir Dis 1971;103: 57–67.

28. Hsu KHK, Jenkins DE, Hsi BP, et al. Ventilatory functions of normal children and young adults: Mexican-American, white, and black. Spirometry. Pediatrics 1979;95:14–23.

29. Schoenberg B, Beck GJ, Bouhuys A. Growth and decay of pulmonary function in healthy blacks and whites. Respir Physiol 1978;33:367–393.

30. Rossiter CE, Weil H. Ethnic differences in lung function: evidence for proportional differences. Int J Epidem 1974;3: 55–61.

31. Stinson JM, McPherson GL, Hicks K, et al. Spirometric standards for healthy black adults. J Nat Med Ass 1981;73:729–733.

32. Boggs PB, Stephens AL, Walker RF, et al. Racially specific reference standards for commonly performed spirometric measurements for black and white children, ages 9–18 years. Ann Allergy 1981;47: 273–277.

SELF-ASSESSMENT QUESTIONS

1. All of the following are techniques for determining FRC except:
   a. closed-circuit helium dilution
   b. open-circuit nitrogen washout
   c. single breath nitrogen washout
   d. body plethysmography

2. Which of the following is the most accurate concerning the expiratory reserve volume:

a. the maximum amount of air that can be exhaled from the vital capacity
b. the maximum amount of air that can be exhaled from the tidal volume end-expiratory level
c. the maximum of air that can be inhaled from the tidal volume end-expiratory level
d. the maximum amount of air that can be exhaled from residual volume

3. A patient has the following lung volumes:

	Observed	Predicted	%Predicted
SVC (L)	3.50	4.30	81
FRC (L)	3.80	3.00	127
RV (L)	3.00	2.00	150
TLC (L)	6.50	6.30	103

The interpretation would most likely state:
a. normal lung volumes
b. hyperinflation
c. restrictive pattern
d. mixed obstructive and restrictive pattern

4. In patients with obstructive lung disease, the gas dilution methods for FRC determination:
a. overestimate FRC
b. equal body plethysmograph FRC
c. underestimate FRC
d. equal radiographic FRC

5. In the body plethysmograph, alveolar pressure changes caused by the compression and decompression of the lungs are estimated by:
a. measuring mouth pressure
b. measuring body box pressure
c. measuring transpulmonary pressure
d. measuring transdiaphragmatic pressure

6. The calculation of FRC using the body plethysmograph is based on:
a. Murphy's law
b. Boyle's law
c. Charles' law
d. Poiseuille's law

7. Which of the following methods for determining total lung capacity best agree with the results of the roentgenographic technique in patients with obstructive lung disease:

    a. body box FRC + IC

    b. closed-circuit helium dilution FRC + IC

    c. open-circuit nitrogen washout FRC + IC

    d. open-circuit helium dilution FRC + IC

8. Which of the following is most accurate about the FRC?

    a. It is the volume of air remaining in the lungs at tidal volume end-expiratory level.

    b. It consists of residual volume and expiratory reserve volume.

    c. It can be determined by gas dilution and body plethysmography.

    d. all of above

    e. a and c

9. In restrictive lung disease, which lung volume compartment is not decreased?

    a. vital capacity

    b. functional residual capacity

    c. total lung capacity

    d. inspiratory capacity

    e. none of above

10. In obstructive lung disease, the slow vital capacity will probably be:

    a. larger than the total lung capacity

    b. smaller than the residual volume

    c. larger than the forced vital capacity

    d. smaller than the inspiratory capacity

3

Single Breath Carbon Monoxide Diffusing Capacity

The process of diffusion is defined as the flow of particles from an area of higher concentration to an area of lower concentration. The measurement of diffusion, as performed in pulmonary function laboratories, provides information about the transfer of gas between the alveoli and the pulmonary capillary blood and is referred to as the **diffusing capacity**. Europeans prefer the term "transfer factor" because the term "diffusing capacity" is somewhat misleading for two reasons: (*a*) Many factors in addition to diffusing characteristics affect the outcome of this test, and (*b*) the outcome of the test is related to metabolic rate and the test is usually done at rest; thus, the outcome is submaximal and, therefore, not a capacity. However, I will use "diffusing capacity" because it is the most commonly used term in the United States.

Measurement of diffusing capacity using carbon monoxide can be performed using three general techniques: (*a*) **steady state,** (*b*) **rebreathing**, and (*c*) **single breath.** Because the focus of this book is on commonly performed tests, only the single breath technique will be discussed.

The single breath carbon monoxide diffusing capacity (DLCO or also denoted as DLCO$_{sb}$) was first measured by Marie and August Krogh in 1914.[1] Forster and coworkers[2] described a modification of Krogh's technique and used helium as a tracer gas in the inspired gas mixture that allowed for the measurement of the dilution of the inspired gas into the lung residual volume.

Over the years, many controversies developed, including how to measure breathhold time, correction for hemoglobin, inspired oxygen pressure, and adjustment for carboxyhemoglobin, carbon dioxide absorption, and valve dead space. In a recent statement,[3] the American Thoracic Society (ATS) addressed these and other problems. This statement has resulted in better technique standardization and improved quality of results.

PHYSIOLOGY

The diffusion of gases in the lungs occurs between alveoli and pulmonary capillary blood. The two major gases involved in lung diffusion (oxygen and carbon dioxide) must move through two barriers: (*a*) alveolar-capillary (A-C) membrane and (*b*) the blood plasma–red blood cell barrier.

The rate of diffusion across these primarily liquid barriers is limited by (*a*) the surface area for diffusion, (*b*) the distance the gas molecules must travel, (*c*) the solubility coefficient of the gases in liquid, (*d*) the partial pressure difference (gradient) between air and blood for each gas, and (*e*) the density of each gas.

Oxygen and carbon dioxide are more soluble in blood than in the A-C membrane and have a strong affinity for hemoglobin. But because these gases are found in venous blood, they are not suitable for the measurement of diffusion capacity. Carbon monoxide (CO) is more advantageous than other gases because of the following characteristics: It has a great affinity for hemoglobin (210 times that of oxygen), it is soluble in blood, and its concentration in venous blood is insignificant. Although CO can be toxic if it combines with a large amount of hemoglobin, it is not dangerous in low concentrations. Thus, the measurement of carbon monoxide diffusing capacity involves the rate of consumption (uptake) of CO by the blood, from the alveoli.

The diffusion or transfer of CO from alveoli to hemoglobin can be separated into four components: (*a*) diffusion across the A-C membrane, (*b*) transfer to the red blood cell, (*c*) passage through the red blood cell membrane, and (*d*) the CO-hemoglobin reaction rate.

The rate of diffusion of a gas across the A-C membrane (Dm) depends on (*a*) the difference between the gas tension (or partial pressure) in the alveolus and in the plasma, (*b*) surface area available for diffusion, (*c*) distance the gas molecules must travel, and (*d*) characteristic of the tissue. Thus, Dm will be altered or decreased when there is increased interstitial fluid, increased fibrotic tissue, increased interalveolar fluid, mismatching of perfused capillaries and ventilated alveoli, pulmonary emboli, or poor ventilation.

The transfer to the red blood cell is dependent on the volume of red blood cells in the pulmonary capillary bed (Qc). Thus, Qc will be altered by position, exercise, and pulmonary circulation.

The passage through the red blood cell membrane and combination with the hemoglobin molecule (Θ_{co}) are the final two processes that complete the diffusion of a gas from alveolus to hemoglobin molecule.

The relationship of these components can be expressed as follows:

$$\frac{1}{DL} = \frac{1}{Dm} + \frac{1}{\Theta Qc}$$

where DL is the diffusing capacity of the lung, Dm is the diffusing capacity of the A-C membrane, Θ is the reaction rate of the gas with the hemoglobin molecule, and Qc is the volume of blood in the alveolar capillaries.

The diffusing capacity of the lung (DL) for carbon monoxide (CO) is the rate of uptake of CO per minute ($\dot{V}_{co}$) per mean gradient of CO across the A-C membrane. This can be stated mathematically as:

$$DLCO = \frac{\dot{V}_{co}}{PA_{co} - Pc_{co}} \text{ ml/min/mm Hg}$$

Where: DLCO = diffusing capacity of the lung for carbon monoxide; $\dot{V}_{co}$ = carbon monoxide uptake from the alveolar gas to the blood per minute; PA_{co} = mean alveolar carbon monoxide pressure; Pc_{co} = mean capillary carbon monoxide pressure.

Three general techniques for measuring the diffusing capacity of the lung are **steady state, rebreathing,** and **single breath.**

There are several steady-state techniques, including the Filey method, end-tidal CO method, and assumed dead space method. These techniques are infrequently used as clinical tests and more commonly used to answer research questions. The rebreathing technique is rarely used because of technique and computation complexity.

The single breath method is the most commonly used technique. The patient first empties his/her lungs, then inhales as deeply as possible a gas mixture (containing carbon monoxide, an inert gas such as helium or neon, and air), and then holds his/her breath for approximately 10 seconds. After this, the patient exhales, and a sample of gas is collected and analyzed for CO and helium. Although this method is quick and does not require blood samples, it is criticized because it measures diffusing capacity at maximal inspiration and during breathholding—neither of which is a "normal" breathing state. A newer technique[4] that requires a maximal inspiration but eliminates the breathhold may be beneficial in the future.

The formula applied for the single breath technique is:

$$DLCO = VA_{STPD} \times \frac{60}{t} \times \frac{1}{PB - 47} \times \ln \frac{FACO_o}{FACO_t}$$

Where: DLCO = diffusing capacity of the lung for CO expressed in ml/min/ mm Hg; VA_{STPD} = the lung volume to which the CO was distributed and determined by:

$$VA_{STPD} = VI_{STPD} \times \frac{FIHe}{FAHe}$$

Where: VI_{STPD} = inspired volume at STPD in milliliters (ml); FIHe = inspired helium concentration; FAHe = alveolar or expired helium concentration; $FACO_o$ = alveolar concentration of CO at start of test and expressed by:

$$\frac{FAHe}{FIHe} \times FICO$$

Where: FAHe = alveolar or expired helium concentration; FIHe = inspired helium concentration; FICO = inspired CO concentration; $FACO_t$ = alveolar concentration of CO at end of test, which is equivalent to the concentration of CO in the expired sample; t = breathhold time (in seconds); 60 = conversion to minutes; PB − 47 = barometric pressure minus water vapor pressure at 37°C; ln = natural logarithm.

INSTRUMENTATION

The technique described by Ogilvie and colleagues,[5] which has become known as the **"classic" technique**, uses a closed-circuit bag-in-box connected to a spirometer as shown in Figure 3.1. The patient is attached to a valve that allows him/her to breathe from one of four circuits (thus, it is sometimes called a 4-way valve). The technician manually turns the valve to connect the patient to the desired circuit.

Two gases are used with the classic technique: (*a*) an inert gas such as helium and (*b*) carbon monoxide. They are analyzed by specific analyzers connected to the system.

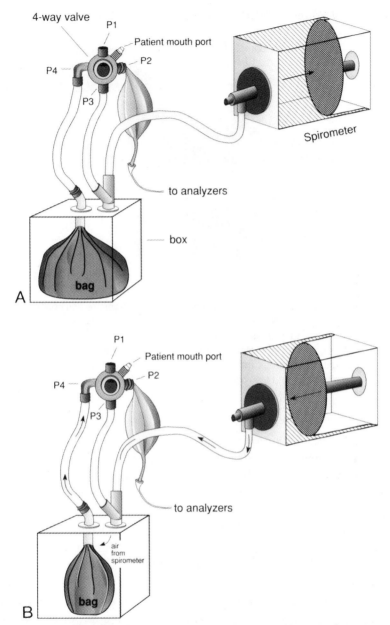

Figure 3.1. Closed-circuit bag-in-box system with connections to spirometer and 4-way valve. In **A**, the bag (sometimes called "balloon") holds the inspired gas mixture. The 4-way valve connects the patient mouth port to one of four openings: (a) P_1 is to room air, (b) P_2 is to the alveolar sample bag, (c) P_3 is to the box, (d) P_4 is from the inspired gas sample. Only one opening can be used at any one time, thus if the patient inhales the gas mixture through P_4, the other openings are closed. When the patient inhales the gas mixture, the bag volume decreases, causing a negative pressure inside the box (but outside the bag). A volume of air equal to the quantity inhaled and contained in the spirometer then enters the box equalizing the pressure as shown in **B**. This volume change in the spirometer is measured to determine the inspired volume by the patient.

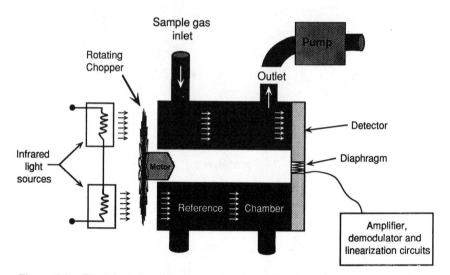

Figure 3.2. The infrared analyzer is commonly used to measure gas concentrations of CO_2, CO, N_2O, and others. It operates by emitting infrared light aimed toward a detector cell. The light passes through a rotating chopper blade, which causes a "pulsed" pattern, which helps stabilize the circuit. As specific gas molecules absorb the infrared light, the detector measures the differences between the reference and gas sample chambers, and the results are sent to amplifiers and linearization circuits.

There are several types of CO analyzers: infrared absorption, electrochemical cell, gas chromatograph, and mass spectrometer. The most practical and most commonly used type in the DLCO testing systems is the **infrared CO analyzer**, and the measuring technique is that of infrared absorption. Simply put, two identical infrared beams are directed through two parallel chambers (Fig. 3.2). One chamber contains a known gas and is referred to as the "reference chamber." The second chamber contains the sample or unknown gas. The infrared beams pass through the chambers and are directed to a single detector unit that converts the beams to an electronic signal.

The major criticism of the infrared absorption CO analyzer is its alinearity characteristic. The problem arises from the fact that two molecules of gas can exist in the sample gas chamber, one directly behind the other. The molecule closest to the infrared light source absorbs the light, but the second molecule does not. Thus, there can be more molecules of gas (i.e., a higher concentration) than is shown. However, most manufacturers have solved this problem by passing the output signal through a linearizing network.

Helium analyzers are the same type used in the devices that determine functional residual capacity (FRC) by helium dilution. They operate on the thermal conductivity principle, which is based on the fact that gases are able to conduct heat—different gases conduct at different rates. Introducing gas molecules into a sampling chamber containing a heated wire causes the temperature of that wire to decrease, allowing more current to flow. In order to be specific for helium, other gases (e.g., carbon dioxide and nitrogen) either must be removed or must be compared to a reference.

The classic technique uses a spirometer connected to the bag-in-box to measure volume. The type of spirometer can vary (e.g., water-seal, rolling-seal). Some of the modified classic techniques sold by vendors employ a pneumotach and use integrated flow to measure volume.

As with other pulmonary function tests, calibration is very important. The spirometers or flow meters (pneumotachs) should be calibrated with a known-volume syringe, and the timing mechanism should be checked against a stopwatch and adjusted if necessary.

Because the calculation of the diffusing capacity is based on examining the changes in the concentrations of the two gases, the analyzers must be linear. Because infrared CO analyzers are nonlinear, it is very important that they be linearized by the laboratory or by the manufacturer. Helium analyzers are linear and usually do not require linearization conditioning.

The test gas should contain the following, accurately analyzed to the level shown in parentheses:

1. 0.3% carbon monoxide ($\pm 0.05\%$)
2. 10.0% helium ($\pm 1\%$), or other inert gas such as neon
3. 21% oxygen ($\pm 2\%$)

The recommendation of 21% oxygen in the test gas applies to sea level. Laboratories at altitudes other than sea level have two alternatives: (*a*) increase the oxygen concentration to produce a PIO_2 of 150 mm Hg [where $PIO_2 = (PB - 47) \times FIO_2$], or (*b*) use an oxygen concentration of 21% regardless of altitude and adjust the results, if necessary, as part of the interpretation.[3] One simple equation that can be used to adjust the DLCO for interpretative purposes only is:

Altitude Adjusted DLCO =
$$\text{Measured DLCO} \times [1.0 + 0.0031 (PIO_2 - 150)]$$

where: $PIO_2 = 0.21 (PB - 47)$

TECHNIQUE

The ATS recommendations[3] for a standardized technique for the single breath carbon monoxide diffusing capacity test (DLCO) were published in 1987.* Since then, many laboratories and vendors have adopted these recommendations, and the technique that I describe is based largely on those recommendations.

Patient Preparation

Patients should be asked to refrain from smoking for 24 hours before the test, since smoking raises the blood carbon monoxide or carboxyhemoglobin level, which is sometimes referred to as **CO back pressure**.

Sympathomimetic bronchodilators may increase the DLCO. In unpublished work, I have shown that inhaled sympathomimetic bronchodilators increase the DLCO values for up to 30 minutes after inhalation. Therefore, I recommend that the DLCO be done before bronchodilator administration or at least 30 minutes after.

Basic Maneuver

Patients, attached to the mouthpiece, wearing noseclips, seated comfortably, and breathing normal tidal volume breaths, should be coached to:

1. Slowly exhale to maximum expiratory level (residual volume);
2. Quickly inhale the analyzed test gas to maximum inhalation level (total lung capacity—an inspiratory vital capacity);
3. Breathhold for approximately 10 seconds;
4. Exhale at a moderate speed after the breathhold;
5. Continue exhaling while technicians collect a sample of exhaled gas, called the "alveolar gas sample";
6. Remove the mouthpiece and rest while technicians analyze the alveolar gas sample;
7. Repeat the procedure until at least two acceptable tests have been obtained (that agree within 10% or 3 ml/min/mm Hg, whichever is larger), allowing at least 4 minutes to elapse between trials.

The ATS recommendations[3] that apply to this basic maneuver are:

---

*The ATS recommendations are for the "classic" bag-in-box system in which a separate alveolar gas sample is collected and helium is used as the inert gas. Manufacturers of systems that use different inert gases other than helium (e.g., neon), or gas sources (e.g., demand valves), flow sensors, or different gas analyzers must demonstrate that their modifications do not alter DLCO when compared to the traditional bag-in-box system values.[3]

1. The inspired vital capacity of test gas should be at least 90% of the largest previously measured vital capacity. The rate of inspiration should be rapid and the inspired volume should be inhaled in less than 4 seconds.
2. The breathhold should last between 9 and 11 seconds, and patients should relax against the closed glottis or valve, avoiding excessive positive or negative intrathoracic pressure.
3. The initial volume of gas exhaled after the breathhold is discarded because it contains gas that resided in the conducting airways. This washout volume should be 750 to 1000 ml if patients' vital capacities are >2 liters. If their vital capacities are <2 liters, the washout volume may be reduced to 500 ml.
4. The volume of the alveolar gas sample should be 500 to 1000 ml and should be collected within 3 seconds.

Practical Hints

In the laboratory, the DLCO test can be performed before other tests, in between other tests, or after the other tests. I recommend that the DLCO test be performed after spirometry or lung volume determinations for two reasons: (*a*) The DLCO maneuver is somewhat more complicated to perform for patients than other pulmonary function tests and, thus, successful completion of the DLCO test is accomplished faster and with fewer attempts if done after other pulmonary function tests, and (*b*) the spirometric results also provide information for the technician as to what vital capacity was achieved and, thus, what the 90% target volume should be.

In cases where patients have severe airflow limitation, after-bronchodilator DLCO measurements might be more successful than before-bronchodilator measurements. In some cases where a significant response to a bronchodilator has occurred, before and after DLCO measurements can be useful. If performing after-bronchodilator DLCO measurements, remember that β-agonists can increase heart rate and cardiac output and, thus, can affect the DLCO value.

The amount of hemoglobin available has an effect on the outcome of a DLCO test. The more hemoglobin available, the higher the DLCO value, and the less hemoglobin available, the lower the DLCO value. Thus, the correction for hemoglobin is an essential part of the calculation process. Therefore, I recommend that a hemoglobin value be obtained on each patient having a DLCO test. Unless the patient has serious bleeding problems, a hemoglobin value obtained within 7 to 10 days should be adequate.

CALCULATIONS

The basic formula for the calculation of the single breath carbon monoxide diffusing capacity (DLCO) of the lung is:

$$\text{DLCO} = \text{VA}_{\text{STPD}} \times \frac{60}{t} \times \frac{1}{PB - 47} \times \ln \frac{\text{FACO}_o}{\text{FACO}_t}$$

Where: VA_{STPD} = alveolar volume at STPD; 60 = conversion to minutes; $PB - 47$ = barometric pressure minus water vapor pressure at 37°C; ln = natural logarithm; FACO_o = fractional concentration of CO in alveoli at start of test; FACO_t = fractional concentration of CO in alveoli at end of test.

This basic equation can be simplified into the following:

$$\text{DLCO} = \frac{\text{VA}_{\text{STPD}} \times 60}{(PB - 47) \times t} \times \ln \left[\frac{\text{He}_E}{\text{He}_I} \times \frac{\text{CO}_I}{\text{CO}_E} \right]$$

Where: VA_{STPD} = volume inspired at ATPD $\times \dfrac{\text{He}_I}{\text{He}_E} \times$ (ATPD to STPD factor); He_E = expired helium concentration after breathhold; He_I = inspired helium concentration; CO_I = inspired carbon monoxide concentration; CO_E = expired carbon monoxide concentration after breathhold.

Example: Calculation of DLCO

A 45-year-old man performs a DLCO test. His hemoglobin is 15.7 g/DL and he claims to be a nonsmoker. The following data are obtained from the test:

Barometric pressure = 729 mm Hg
Volume inspired = 5130 ml at 23°C
Helium inspired = 10.0
Carbon monoxide inspired = 0.309
Helium expired = 7.3
Carbon monoxide expired = 0.102
Breathhold time = 10.7 sec

Calculate the DLCO. The DLCO can be calculated in two steps:
STEP 1: Calculate the alveolar volume.

$$\text{VA}_{\text{STPD}} = \text{volume inspired at ATPD} \times \frac{\text{He}_I}{\text{He}_E} \times (\text{ATPD to STPD factor})$$

$$\text{VA}_{\text{STPD}} = 5130 \times \frac{10.0}{7.3} \times 0.8847$$

$$\text{VA}_{\text{STPD}} = 6217 \text{ ml at STPD}$$

STEP 2: Calculate the DLCO

$$DLCO = \frac{VA_{STPD} \times 60}{(PB - 47) \times t} \times \ln \left[\frac{He_E}{He_I} \times \frac{CO_I}{CO_E} \right]$$

$$DLCO = \frac{6217 \times 60}{(729 - 47) \times 10.7} \times \ln \left[\frac{7.3}{10.0} \times \frac{0.309}{0.102} \right]$$

$$DLCO = \frac{373,020}{7,297} \times \ln 2.2115$$

$$DLCO = 51.12 \times 0.7937$$

$$DLCO = 40.57 \text{ ml/min/mm Hg}$$

The ATS Statement recommendations include:

1. **Breathhold time:** Either the classic Ogilvie technique[5] (beginning of inspiration to beginning of alveolar gas sample collection) or the Jones-Meade tech-

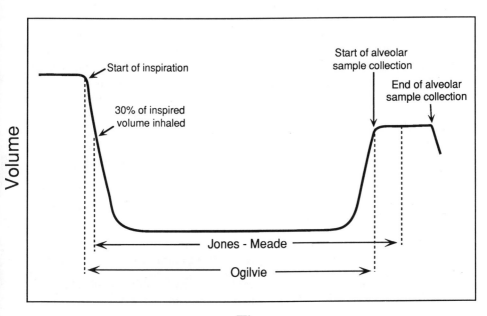

Figure 3.3. Graphic illustration of the two recommended methods for measuring the breathhold time for the single breath DLCO. The Ogilvie or "classic" method starts the breathhold time from the beginning of inspiration of the test gas and ends the breathhold time at the beginning of the alveolar sample collection. The Jones-Meade method starts the breathhold time after 30% of the test gas has been inhaled, and ends the breathhold time halfway into the alveolar sample collection.

nique[6] (which starts after 30% of the inspired volume has been inhaled, and ends when 50% of the alveolar gas sample has been collected) should be used. A third technique[7] has been used but is not recommended by the ATS. The two recommended methods for calculating breathhold time are shown in Figure 3.3.

2. **Inspired volume (V_I) dead space:** Adjustments should be made for instrument (usually 100 ml) and anatomic dead space (approximately 150 ml) and subtracted from the measured V_I.

3. **CO_2 absorption:** When CO_2 is absorbed prior to gas analysis, the expired helium and CO concentrations are artifactually increased, thus decreasing the true alveolar volume. If the alveolar CO_2 concentration is assumed to be 5%, the correction would be $1.05 \times VA$ (1% for each percent of alveolar CO_2).

4. **Hemoglobin concentration:** DLCO changes as a function of hemoglobin concentration and, therefore, it is recommended that the measured DLCO be hemoglobin adjusted using the technique of Cotes.[8]

$$\text{Hemoglobin Corrected DLCO} = \text{Observed DLCO} \times \frac{(10.22 + Hb)}{(1.7 \times Hb)}$$

This correction assumes a standard hemoglobin of 14.6. Thus, DLCO values in patients with hemoglobin values higher than 14.6 g/DL will be lowered after adjustment. Conversely, the DLCO values in patients with hemoglobin values lower than 14.6 g/DL will be higher after adjustment. The ATS recommendation is always report to the uncorrected DLCO value, even if the hemoglobin-adjusted DLCO is also reported.

5. **Carboxyhemoglobin:** An adjustment for blood CO levels is not required. However, if an adjustment is made, the recommendation is that the DLCO is increased by 1% for each percent of carboxyhemoglobin. The following formula can be used:

$$CO_{Hb} \text{ corrected DLCO} = \text{measured DLCO} \times \left(1 + \frac{\% \ CO_{Hb}}{100} \right)$$

Other Calculations and Adjustments

The alveolar volume (VA_{STPD}) measured during the DLCO test includes the anatomical and mechanical (i.e., valve) dead space. The ATS recommendation[3] is to subtract these two dead space volumes (totaling approximately 200 to 300 ml) from the inspired volume.

When VA_{STPD} is converted to VA_{BTPS} (which is how it should be reported), even when anatomical dead space has been subtracted, the result is an approximation of total lung capacity measured by a single breath helium (or other inert gas) equilibration technique. The comparison of VA_{BTPS} to total lung capacity (by other lung volume measurement methods, which

I refer to as TLC_{om}) in healthy individuals in my laboratory is very good (i.e., $VA_{BTPS}/TLC_{om} = 0.90 - 1.05$).

As can be seen from the mathematical formula, alveolar volume (VA) is a critical component of the DLCO value. As VA increases, the DLCO will increase, and as VA decreases, the DLCO will decrease. Because of this relationship, the ratio of diffusing capacity and alveolar volume ($DLCO/VA_{BTPS}$) is commonly reported.

QUALITY CONTROL

Calculation of the DLCO value involves the manipulation of data from several components. Therefore, quality control for the DLCO test can be approached from two avenues: (*a*) Quality control the components individually, and/or (*b*) quality control the components collectively.

The individual components consist of:

1. **Gas analyzers:** These must be linear because the calculation uses the ratio of the two helium concentrations (i.e., He_I/He_E) and the ratio of the two CO concentrations (i.e., CO_I/CO_E). The ATS recommends[3] CO infrared analyzer linearity checks at least every 6 months, and I recommend linearity checks of the helium analyzer every 12 months.
2. **Timing device:** Small changes in breathhold time (e.g., 0.5 to 1.0 sec) can cause large changes in the DLCO value. Therefore, the timing device must be accurate and should be checked every 3 months.[9]
3. **Volume measuring device:** A calibration syringe should be used daily to calibrate the volume measuring system. If volume displacement spirometers are used, leak testing is also necessary.

It is important that the dead space of the system be known and that the CO_2 and H_2O absorbers be fresh and be positioned so that gas passes through them before entering the analyzers.

The two collective quality-control checks that I recommend for the DLCO system are (*a*) alveolar volume check and (*b*) DLCO measured in laboratory standards.

The **alveolar volume check** ensures that the volume-measuring device and helium analyzer are correct. I recommend this be done every 3 months. Connect a syringe of known volume (e.g., 3 liters) to the patient port of the valve with minimal space between syringe and port. With the syringe partially empty (e.g., in a 3-liter syringe set at 2 liters, thus 1 liter has been ejected), withdraw enough test gas to fill the syringe. Wait approximately 5 to 10 seconds and eject enough volume to satisfy dead space clearance requirements and to obtain an "alveolar" sample of adequate volume. The helium concentration before and after this maneuver and volume inspired by the syringe can be used to calculate the expected VA (the volume of the syringe—3 liters in the example just used). The formula for calculating the known VA is the same as the one used to calculate VA during patient testing, except temperature correction is not done:

$$VA = VI \times \frac{HE_I}{He_E} - \text{(valve and set-up dead space)}$$

Where: VA = expected syringe volume; VI = volume inspired using syringe; HE_I = initial helium concentration; He_E = final helium concentration.

Let's use an example to illustrate the use of this method. A 3-liter syringe is attached to the patient port of the DLCO system with a rubber connector. The valve and connector dead space is 200 ml. The syringe is set so that it contains 1 liter (i.e., one-third full) and is connected to the patient port of the DLCO system. This mimics a patient with a 1-liter residual volume (RV) and a 2-liter vital capacity (VC). Thus the VA (RV + VC) is approximately 3 liters, which is the value we are trying to achieve. Withdraw 2 liters of test gas, thereby filling the syringe, and pause approximately 5 to 10 seconds and then eject 500 ml before collecting an alveolar sample. The following data are obtained: inspired vital capacity VI_{ATPD} = 2.0 liters; initial helium reading (He_I) = 9.95; final helium reading (He_E) = 6.11; dead space (valve + connector) = 200 ml (0.2 liters).

$$VA = VI \times \frac{He_I}{He_E} - \text{(valve and set-up dead space)}$$

$$VA = 2.0 \times \frac{9.95}{6.11} - 0.2$$

$$VA = 3.26 - 0.2$$

VA = 3.06 liters at ATPD (since a room temperature syringe was used)

I use a ±3% checking criterion, and therefore the range of acceptability in this example would be 2.91 to 3.09 liters. Thus, the system used is accurately determining alveolar volume.

The use of **laboratory standards** (healthy, nonsmoking individuals) in the pulmonary function laboratory is widespread and is the second collective method for quality controlling the DLCO system. Although it does not provide an absolute value, it does provide a value that remains reasonably constant over time, which allows the laboratory personnel to detect changes. The ATS recommends DLCO testing on laboratory standards at least twice a month. If a standard subject's measured DLCO value varies by more than 11% from his/her average DLCO value, the system should be considered "out of control" and the individual components of the system should be carefully evaluated.[3]

BASIC ELEMENTS OF INTERPRETATION

Examination of Reference Studies

As with other pulmonary function values, the DLCO is compared to reference values generated from studies on healthy populations. Many such studies have been published and there are differences. For example, if the reference or predicted DLCO value is calculated for a 45-year-old male, 68 inches (173 cm) tall using the reference equations of Crapo,[10] Paoletti,[11] Knudson,[12] Cotes,[13] and Miller,[14] the following results are obtained:

Study	DLCO
Cotes	29.62 ml/min/mm Hg
Crapo	35.77
Paoletti	36.20
Knudson	37.75
Miller	31.03

Unfortunately, the variability of these reference values is large. One likely reason is the variations in technique.

While the reference equations for these studies are listed in Table 3.1, the reader should know more about how each study was carried out. Therefore, let us scrutinize these studies.

The equations published by Cotes[13] in his first edition (1965) of *Lung Function* were from unpublished work, and little is known about the methods.

Crapo and Morris's reference values (published in 1981)[10] are widely used. Their study used a bag-in-box technique with helium as the inert gas. The breathhold time was calculated using the technique of Ogilvie (beginning of inspiration to the beginning of alveolar gas sample collection). They used 25% oxygen in the inspired gas sample and used the results from 123 men (age range 16 to 91) and 122 women (age range 17 to 84).

Miller and coworkers[14] studied smokers and nonsmokers in their 1983 study. Their method used a demand valve from the tank of inspired gas with a pneumotach instead of the bag-in-box. The breathhold time was cal-

Table 3.1: Reference equations for single breath carbon monoxide diffusing capacity

Cotes[13]:
  Men: DLCO = 32.5 (Htmeters) − 0.2 (age) − 17.6
  Women: DLCO = 21.2 (Htmeters) − 0.156 (age) − 2.66

Crapo[10]:
  Men:
    DLCO uncorrected for Hb = 0.416 (Htcm) − 0.219 (age) − 26.34, SEE = 4.83
    DLCO corrected for Hb = 0.410 (Htcm) − 0.210 (age) − 26.31, SEE = 4.82

  Women:
    DLCO uncorrected for Hb = 0.256 (Htcm) − 0.144 (age) − 8.36, SEE = 3.57
    DLCO corrected for Hb = 0.282 (Htcm) − 0.157 (age) − 10.89, SEE = 3.6

Paoletti[11]:
  Men: 19–65 years: DLCO = 0.4410 (Htcm) − 0.1936 (age) − 31.3822 SEE = 5.79
  Women: 19–65 years: DLCO = 0.1569 (Htcm) − 0.0677 (age) + 5.0767 SEE = 4.31

Knudson[12]:
  Men <25: DLCO = 0.328 (Htcm) + 0.722 (age) − 30.9685, SEE = 3.97
  Men ≥25: DLCO = 0.3551 (Htcm) − 0.2741 (age) − 11.3527, SEE = 4.57
  Women <20: DLCO = 0.3808 (Htcm) − 32.9232, SEE = 3.52
  Women ≥20: DLCO = 0.1872 (Htcm) − 0.146 (age) + 3.8821, SEE = 4.50

Miller[14]:
  Men: DLCO = 0.418 (Htin) − 0.229 (age) + 12.911
  Women: DLCO = 0.4068 (Htin) − 0.1111 (age) + 2.238

culated using the technique recommended by the Epidemiology Standardization Project (ESP)[7]—when half of the inspired vital capacity has been inhaled, to the beginning of alveolar gas sample collection. The average of two tests was reported, and there were 74 men nonsmokers and 130 women nonsmokers.

Paoletti and coworkers[11] studied the general population of the Po river delta near Venice, Italy, in 1985. An automated demand valve system with a pneumotach was used. The breathhold time was calculated using the ESP technique.[7] There were 163 men in the age range of 8 to 19, and 80 men in the age range of 19 to 65. There were 178 women in the age range of 8 to 18, and 291 women in the age range of 19 to 65. The inspired gas contained 20% oxygen.

Knudson and coworkers[12] studied a non-Mexican-American population in Tucson, Arizona, from 1981 to 1984. A commercially modified bag-in-box system was used—a double water-sealed spirometer. The inert gas was helium, and 21% oxygen was used in the inspired gas. The breathhold time was calculated using the ESP technique.[7] There were 28 men under age 25 and 71 men over age 25. There were 30 women under 20 years of age and 99 women over 20 years of age.

Choosing a Reference Equation

When selecting reference equations for your laboratory, know the methodology and try to choose a study that used techniques similar to the ones you use. Likewise, choose a study that used a population that is similar to your patient population. Also, examine the number of patients in the age range reported by the study. Choose one or two "candidate" studies that match as many criteria as possible with your laboratory; then, measure the DLCO in 10 to 15 healthy nonsmoking individuals and compare the results to the predicted or reference values from the candidate reference studies. If the difference between the measured DLCO value and the reference value is zero, the reference equation "fits" the laboratory population. The best equation is the one that produces the smallest difference between calculated and measured values in healthy subjects.

Lower Limit of Normal

The lower limit of normal is controversial. Some clinicians[15] use the 95th percentile obtained by multiplying the standard error of estimate (SEE) of the regression equation by 1.64 and subtracting that value from the mean reference value. Other clinicians use 80 or 85% of the reference value as the lower limit of normal.

Decreased DLCO

Once the lower limit of normal has been determined for your laboratory, low DLCO values can be identified. Additionally, because alveolar volume is also determined, the ratio DLCO/VA can be applied and is useful in evaluating the causes of a reduced DLCO.

A good example of decreased DLCO is in patients with emphysema. In these patients, the loss of alveolar-capillary bed as alveoli rupture results in reduced surface area available for diffusion. The alveolar volume in which the CO was distributed is often of normal size or increased, and, thus, the DLCO/VA is reduced. In these situations (i.e., low DLCO and low DLCO/VA), the interpretation should simply state that a low DLCO is observed.

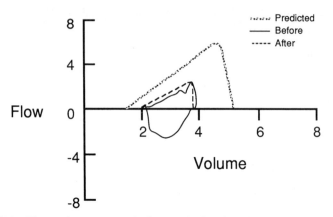

Figure 3.4. Flow volume curves before and after bronchodilator on 56-year-old women in Case 3.1. The curves are positioned at absolute lung volume obtained by body plethysmography.

In patients with restrictive processes (e.g., sarcoidosis, scleroderma, chest-wall deformity), the DLCO is also commonly reduced. However, the alveolar volume is also low, resulting in a normal DLCO/VA that suggests that the reduced DLCO is due to small lungs rather than a diffusion abnormality. Therefore, the interpretation should state that a low DLCO value was obtained and that it is normalized when corrected for volume.

CASE 3.1

A 56-year-old white woman who claimed to be a nonsmoker and to have had a pneumonectomy 4 years ago was tested in the pulmonary function laboratory. Her pulmonary function test results are shown in Figure 3.4 and Table 3.2.

Questions
1. What is the interpretation of the pulmonary function data?
2. Is there adequate information for interpreting all the results?

Answers and Discussion
The pulmonary function data can be partially interpreted. The lung volume (as measured by total lung capacity) is decreased. There is also airflow limitation, which does not significantly improve with bronchodilator. These findings would suggest a mixed restrictive and obstructive process.

The DLCO is decreased, but there is not enough information to adequately interpret this finding. In order to accurately interpret the single breath DLCO value, the alveolar volume must be taken into consideration.

Table 3.2: Pulmonary function data before and after bronchodilator on 56-year-old woman in Case 3.1

	Before		After
FVC (L)	1.76	(47)*	1.87
FEV$_1$ (L)	1.22	(42)	1.31
FEV$_1$/FVC (%)	69		70
FEF25-75% (L/sec)	0.80	(27)	0.85
TGV (L)	2.94	(103)	
TLC (L)	3.73	(74)	
RV (L)	1.66	(130)	
DLCO (ml/min/mm Hg)**	14.8	(56)	

* Values in parentheses are percent of predicted
** Corrected for hemoglobin using Cotes[8]

Table 3.3: Single breath carbon monoxide diffusing capacity (DLCO) and DLCO corrected for alveolar volume (DLCO/VA) in 56-year-old woman in Case 3.1

DLCO (ml/min/mm Hg)	14.8	(56)*
DLCO/VA	5.7	(106)**
DLCO/VA	5.7	(110)#

* Values in parentheses are percent of predicted
** Percent predicted using Crapo and Morris[10]
# Percent predicted using predicted TLC divided into predicted DLCO

Because the surface area available for diffusion is dependent on the size of the lungs, the measured DLCO will depend on lung volume. If a patient has only one lung, the DLCO value will be low when compared to a patient with two lungs. Likewise, the DLCO of a patient with one lung will be low when compared to a reference value based on height and age. But if the DLCO is divided by the alveolar volume that the CO was distributed to, the ratio (DLCO/VA) is normal. In this patient, the result of this correction is shown in Table 3.3. Predicted equations for DLCO are available,[10] or the predicted total lung capacity (TLC) could be divided into the predicted DLCO.

If the DLCO is "normal" or greater than normal, correction for alveolar volume is not important. But if the DLCO is low, the DLCO/VA should be considered. In this patient, the measured DLCO is low, but when corrected for alveolar volume, it is normal. This suggests that lung diffusion is normal in the remaining lung.

CASE 3.2

A 21-year-old man who claimed to be a nonsmoker was tested in the pulmonary function laboratory. Results are shown in Table 3.4.

Table 3.4: Pulmonary function data before and after bronchodilator on 21-year-old man in Case 3.2

	Before		After
FVC (L)	4.77	(90)*	4.69
FEV$_1$ (L)	4.21	(102)	4.17
FEV$_1$/FVC (%)	88		89
FEF25-75% (L/sec)	5.13	(110)	5.09
TGV (L)	3.03	(85)	
TLC (L)	5.97	(91)	
RV (L)	1.20	(76)	
DLCO (ml/min/mm Hg)**	32.9	(74)	
DLCO/VA	5.59	(81)	
Arterial Blood Gas			
pH	7.43		
PaCO$_2$ (mm Hg)	39		
PaO$_2$ (mm Hg)	87		
SaO$_2$ (%)	94		
COHb (%)	2.1		
Hb g/DL	10.1		

* Values in parentheses are percent of predicted
** Not corrected for hemoglobin

Question:
How do you interpret the DLCO?

Answer and Discussion:
The spirometry results are normal, and no response to bronchodilator is seen. The lung volumes (TLC, TGV, and RV) are slightly low but still within normal limits.

The DLCO test value is low. When corrected for alveolar volume, it is also low, suggesting a diffusion abnormality. However, the DLCO has not been corrected for hemoglobin. When corrected for hemoglobin, the DLCO becomes 38.9 ml/min/mm Hg, which is 87% of predicted, which is within normal limits.

Carbon monoxide has a very high affinity for hemoglobin. Thus, the diffusion of CO is affected by the amount of hemoglobin in the pulmonary capillaries. Patients with anemia will have low DLCO values because of the low reservoir available for binding with CO. Likewise, patients with polycythemia (increased hemoglobin values) will have high DLCO values because of high reservoirs. Two methods for normalizing the DLCO value to a standard hemoglobin value are widely used.[8,16] The ATS has recommended[3] the use of Cotes's equation,[8] which is:

$$\text{Hemoglobin Corrected DLCO} = \text{Observed DLCO} \times \frac{(10.22 + \text{Hb})}{(1.7 \times \text{Hb})}$$

Table 3.5: Single breath carbon monoxide diffusing capacity values corrected and uncorrected for hemoglobin in 21-year-old male in Case 3.2

Uncorrected DLCO (ml/min/mm Hg)	32.9	(74)*
Corrected DLCO	38.9	(87)
Corrected DLCO/VA	6.60	(95)

* Values in parentheses are percent of predicted

The ATS also states[3] that the uncorrected DLCO always be reported even if the hemoglobin corrected DLCO is also reported as shown in Table 3.5.

REFERENCES

1. Krogh M. The diffusion of gases through the lungs of man. J Physiol 1914; 49: 271–300.
2. Forster RE, Fowler WS, Bates DV, Van Lingen B. The absorption of carbon monoxide by the lungs during breath-holding. J Clin Invest 1954;33:1135–1145.
3. American Thoracic Society Statement. Single breath carbon monoxide diffusing capacity (transfer factor). Am Rev Respir Dis 1987;136:1299–1307.
4. Newth CJL, Cotton DJ, Nadel JA. Pulmonary diffusing capacity measured at multiple intervals during a single exhalation in man. J Appl Physiol 1977;43: 617–625.
5. Ogilvie CM, Forster RE, Blackemore WS, Morton JW. A standardized breath holding technique for the clinical measurement of diffusing capacity of the lung for carbon monoxide. J Clin Invest 1957;36:1–17.
6. Jones RS, Meade F. A theoretical and experimental analysis of anomalies in the estimation of pulmonary diffusing capacity by the single breath method. QJ Exp Physiol 1961;46:131–143.
7. Ferris BG. Epidemiology Standardization Project. Am Rev Respir Dis 1978; (suppl):62–72.
8. Cotes JE. Lung function. 4th ed. London: Blackwell Scientific Publications, 1979.
9. Gardner RM, Clausen JL, Crapo RO, et al. Quality assurance in pulmonary function laboratories. ATS position paper. Am Rev Respir Dis 1986;134:625–627.
10. Crapo RO, Morris AH. Standardized single breath normal values for carbon monoxide diffusing capacity. Am Rev Respir Dis 1981;123:185–189.
11. Paoletti P, Viegi G, Pistelli G, et al. Reference equations for the single breath diffusing capacity. Am Rev Respir Dis 1985; 132:806–813.
12. Knudson RJ, Kaltenborn WT, Knudson DE, Burrows B. The single breath carbon monoxide diffusing capacity. Am Rev Respir Dis 1987;135:805–811.
13. Cotes JE, Lung function: assessment and application in medicine. London: Blackwell Scientific, 1965.
14. Miller A, Thornton JC, Warshaw R, Anderson H, et al. Single breath diffusing capacity in a representative sample of the population of Michigan, a large industrial state. Am Rev Respir Dis 1983; 127:270–277.
15. Crapo RO, Forster RE. Carbon monoxide diffusing capacity. Clin Chest Med 1989;10:187–198.
16. Dinakara P, Blumenthal WS, Johnston RF, Kauffman LA, Solnick PB. The effect of anemia on pulmonary diffusing capacity with derivation of a correction equation. Am Rev Respir Dis 1970;102: 965–969.

SELF-ASSESSMENT QUESTIONS

1. Carbon monoxide has an affinity for hemoglobin that is:
   a. 210 times that of oxygen
   b. 210 times that of carbon dioxide
   c. 2 times that of oxygen
   d. 210 times that of nitrogen

2. All of the following are components of the diffusion or transfer of carbon monoxide from the alveoli to hemoglobin except:
   a. diffusion across the alveolar-capillary membrane
   b. passage through the red blood cell membrane
   c. CO-hemoglobin reaction rate
   d. arterial-alveolar oxygen gradient
   e. transfer to the red blood cell

3. In the single breath DLCO test, an inert gas is included in the inspired gas mixture for the purpose of:
   a. measuring functional residual capacity
   b. measuring the dilution of CO into the lung residual volume
   c. quality control
   d. measuring the diffusion across the A-C membrane

4. In the single breath DLCO test, the alveolar volume is calculated from:
   a. the volume inspired and the dilution of the inert gas
   b. the volume inspired and the dilution of carbon monoxide
   c. the volume inspired and the functional residual capacity
   d. the volume inspired and the dilution of nitrogen

5. The methods of determining breathhold time recommended by the ATS during the single breath DLCO test are:
   I. beginning of inspiration to the beginning of alveolar gas sample collection
   II. after 30% of the inspired volume has been inhaled to 50% of the alveolar gas sample collection time
   III. after 50% of the inspired volume has been inhaled to the beginning of alveolar gas sample collection
   IV. beginning of inspiration to the end of the alveolar gas sample collection
   a. I, IV
   b. I, II

   c. II, III
   d. I, III
   e. III, IV

6. The inspired vital capacity of test gas during the single breath DLCO test should be:
   a. at least 90% of the largest previously measured vital capacity
   b. at least 80% of the largest previously measured vital capacity
   c. inhaled in less than 4 seconds
   d. a and c
   e. b and c

7. Which of the following is true about the alveolar volume (VA_{BTPS}) measured during the single beath DLCO test:
   I. includes the anatomical and valve dead space
   II. includes only the anatomical dead space
   III. is calculated from a single breath helium dilution
   IV. is an approximation of total lung capacity
   a. I only
   b. II only
   c. I, III
   d. I, III, IV
   e. II, III, IV

4

Exercise Tests

The exercise tests performed in the pulmonary function laboratory with which the student and technician should be familiar are of three major types: (*a*) exercise test for exercise-induced asthma, (*b*) exercise tolerance test, and (*c*) exercise test for desaturation using oximetry. This chapter presents these three types of exercise tests in separate sections.

PATIENT SAFETY

A topic that is common to all three types of exercise tests is patient safety. An examination by the attending physician, with a complete review of the patient's history, should precede the ordering of any exercise test.

When the patient arrives in the laboratory, a pretest evaluation should be performed to identify any contraindications. The pretest evaluation should include a preexercise questionnaire, and, in some hospitals, a signed consent form describing the risks and possible discomforts is required. Additionally, the procedure should be carefully explained to the patient.

The pretest evaluation should also include a 12-lead electrocardiogram (EKG) resting blood pressure and in some cases a resting arterial blood gas sample to verify oxygenation status. A doctor should review the questionnaire and results of these tests to determine if any contraindications to exercise are present.[1,2]

Common contraindications to exercise testing

Chest pain
Severe dyspnea
Recent myocardial infarction
Resting hypertension
Ventricular or atrial arrhythmias
Congestive heart failure or aortic valve disease
Severe pulmonary hypertension

A doctor and personnel certified in cardiopulmonary resuscitation (CPR), trained in cardiovascular emergencies, and aware of physiologic changes that occur during exercise should be present or nearby regardless of patient age.

Resuscitation equipment and drugs should be readily available. Additionally, the technician or therapist should have bronchodilators for inhalation, epinephrine, and oxygen available and ready to use.

During the exercise period, blood pressure and breath sounds should be checked periodically, oxygen saturation monitored by oximetry, and the EKG examined continuously to determine if any indications to terminate exercise are present.

Common indications for terminating exercise tests

Severe chest pain with or without ST changes
Severe dyspnea
Dizziness, marked apprehension, or cyanosis
Frequent premature ventricular contractions
Atrial fibrillation
Second- or third-degree heart block, or bundle branch block pattern
Systolic blood pressure above 300 mm Hg, or diastolic blood pressure above 140 mm Hg
Systolic or diastolic blood pressure fall of more than 20 mm Hg after the normal rise with exercise

EXERCISE TEST FOR EXERCISE-INDUCED ASTHMA

It has been recognized for many years that exercise can have adverse effects on the asthmatic patient. As many as 75 to 90% of all asthmatics have exercise-induced asthma (EIA), also called exercise-induced bronchospasm (EIB). Although EIA is especially prevalent in children and adolescents, it affects all age groups.

In the pulmonary function laboratory, the exercise test can be used as a provocation (challenge) tool for the detection of airway hyperresponsiveness. However, unlike methacholine and histamine, it is difficult to study EIA in a dose-response manner because of the physiologic effects of exercise. More commonly, exercise is used to confirm a clinical suspicion of EIA or to evaluate pharmacotherapy.

The purpose of this section is to acquaint the reader with the physiology of exercise in the asthmatic, the preparation of the patient for testing, the pulmonary function tests and testing technique, and basic interpretation.

Physiology

The investigations by Jones and his colleagues[3] in the 1960s pioneered the study of exercise-induced asthma. Although EIA had been recognized previously, Jones and colleagues demonstrated that in asthmatic children:

1. Exercise of 1 to 2 minutes produces an increase in the FEV_1;
2. Prolonged exercise (8 to 12 minutes) produces a decrease in the FEV_1, with the FEV_1 reaching its lowest value 1 to 5 minutes after exercise;
3. Both the increase and decrease can be minimized by pretreatment with a β-sympathomimetic medication.

Since then, other investigators have looked at the effect of duration, type, and intensity of exercise, the refractory period, and the effect of inspired air temperature and water content. Although it is agreed that these factors influence airway response, the exact mechanism of EIA is still unknown.

During an exercise period of 6 to 8 minutes (a standardized time for this test[4]), both the asthmatic and the normal patient have a rise in peak expiratory flow rate (PEFR) and forced expiratory volume in 1 second (FEV_1). It is believed that this bronchodilatation is caused by increased catecholamine release. Near the end of or after the exercise period, the asthmatic patient with EIA has a marked fall in these ventilatory function param-

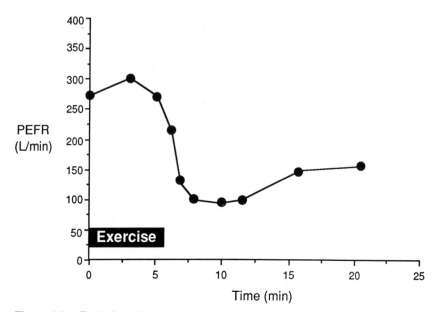

Figure 4.1. Typical ventilatory response (as measured by peak expiratory flow rate) of an asthmatic child to 6 minutes of running. (Modified from Godfrey S, Silverman M, Anderson SD. Problems of interpreting exercise-induced asthma. J Allergy Clin Immunol 1973;52:199–209.)

eters, with the values reaching their lowest level 3 to 15 minutes after exercise (Fig. 4.1).

Running has been reported as being the most asthmogenic form of exercise,[5] with treadmill running being a little less potent than free-running. Cycling is the next most asthmogenic form of exercise, followed by walking, swimming, and kayaking (Fig. 4.2).

The severity of EIA has been shown to depend on the intensity of the exercise.[3,5] The maximum effect occurs when the work rate is approximately 75 to 90% of maximum workload. It is interesting that further increases in intensity beyond this level do not produce more severe EIA.

Two factors that have been shown to play a major role in EIA are heat and water loss from the airway mucosa resulting from increased ventilation. This theory has led to the practice of cooling the inspired air to enhance the bronchospastic response of EIA[6] and to the use of warm, moist, inspired air to reduce the response.[7] If temperature and humidity are factors, one would think that EIA would be more likely to occur and be more severe in drier, colder climates. This has been studied and shown to be true.[8]

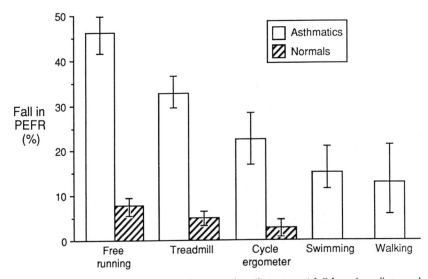

Figure 4.2. Ventilatory response, expressed as the percent fall from baseline peak expiratory flow rate to different types of exercise in groups of asthmatic and normal subjects. The numbers indicate the number of subjects. The bars indicate ±1 standard error of the mean (SEM), and no normal subjects were studied for swimming or treadmill walking. (Modified from Godfrey S, Silverman M, Anderson SD. Problems of interpreting exercise-induced asthma. J Allergy Clin Immunol 1973;52:199–209.)

Heat and moisture loss from the airway mucosa have been shown to influence EIA. However, many investigators believe that other mechanisms also play a role—mechanical stimulation of breathing at a high minute ventilation, lower CO_2 tension, lactic acidosis, stimulation of carotid bodies, release of stored chemical mediators, and imbalance of α- and β-sympathetic discharge.[9,10]

In some patients, both an immediate and a delayed response to EIA are seen, with the late or delayed response occurring 3 to 5 hours after the exercise period.[11] However, the delayed response is uncommon, does not appear to be dependent on the existence of an immediate response, and is not specifically related to exercise.[12,13]

After the exercise period and resulting EIA, a refractory period of 3 to 4 hours occurs.[14,15] During this refractory period, a second exercise period occurring shortly after recovery from the initial exercise will produce an episode of EIA less severe than the first.

Oxygen saturation in patients with EIA follows the pattern of the ventilatory function. During the first few minutes of exercise, there is usually an increase in arterial oxygen tension, and saturation usually occurs. As the flow rates decrease toward the end of or following exercise, oxygen tension and saturation usually fall.[16]

Patient Preparation

The patient should be as drug free as possible for this exercise test because we are trying to determine whether exercise is a trigger for bronchospasm. Inhaled β-sympathomimetic agents (e.g., isoproterenol, metaproterenol, albuterol, terbutaline, and fenoterol), disodium cromoglycate, atropine, antihistamines, and oral and inhaled steroids have been shown to lessen or prevent EIA. However, the oral β-sympathomimetics and theophylline do not prevent EIA, although they do produce significant bronchodilatation.[17]

It is frequently impossible or inadvisable for patients with difficult to control asthma to have some or all of these drugs withheld for long periods of time. In some cases, a patient may be able to avoid bronchodilators for no more than 4 to 6 hours. Such patients (because of the severity of their asthma) usually develop EIA despite taking medications. Thus, a practical yet effective approach is to withhold the following medications prior to the test for the noted time.

Drug	Hours to Withhold
Aerosolized β-sympathomimetics	4–8
Disodium cromoglycate	8
Atropine	8
Antihistamines (short-acting)	24
Antihistamines (long-acting)	72
Inhaled steroids	8

In addition to withholding medications, the patient should also avoid heavy exercise for 4 hours before the test.

The patient should be dressed appropriately for walking or running, with proper footwear such as sneakers or running or walking shoes. Comfortable pants or shorts and a shirt that allows for easy EKG-lead application are also recommended.

Every patient, prior to exercise, should have been examined by a physician who has obtained a thorough history and been able to judge the patient's cardiovascular status. Contraindications for exercise challenges include a history of myocardial infarction or anginalike chest pain, hypertension, or EKG abnormalities.

The preexercise spirometry values should be at least 70% of the patient's best previous prebronchodilator values, with an FEV_1 of at least 1.5 liters. In children, the FEV_1 should be at least 65% of the predicted value. If a patient cannot meet these spirometric criteria, the exercise test should be rescheduled and the medication withholding schedule modified.

Pulmonary Function Tests

The most commonly used pulmonary function test (PFT) used with EIA procedures is forced spirometry. It should be performed according to American Thoracic Society (ATS) recommendations as described in Chapter 1. However, peak flow meters were widely used in many of the early papers and remain a good tool for assessing EIA.

The use of the body plethysmograph to measure specific conductance (SGaw) is sometimes preferred because it does not require a deep breath or a forced expiration and is less effort dependent. However, its use may be impractical, more costly, or not available in many laboratories. Usually, a specified percent fall in FEV_1, PEFR, or SGaw is used to quantify EIA. This is calculated in the following way:

$$\% \text{ Fall} = \frac{\text{Preexercise value} - \text{Postexercise value}}{\text{Preexercise value}} \times 100$$

The PFT should be performed before exercise, with repetition until good reproducibility is obtained. The result should be evaluated to assure that function is adequate for testing as noted above. The PFTs should be repeated at approximately 3 to 5 minutes after exercise, and if EIA is not apparent, PFTs should be repeated 10 to 15 minutes after exercise is terminated.

The specific decrease in PEFR or FEV_1 necessary to be interpreted as EIA is controversial. However, two sources suggest that a fall in FEV_1 or PEFR of at least 10% should be considered positive for EIA.[18,19] Table 4.1 classifies the percent fall in FEV_1 or PEFR by severity.[20] When SGaw is used to diagnose EIA, a fall $\geq 40\%$ is required for a positive diagnosis.

Testing Technique

The purpose of the exercise test is to demonstrate the presence of a meaningful decrease in ventilatory function following exercise.

The treadmill is the recommended mode of exercise. Although free-running is more asthmogenic, it has shortcomings as an EIA-testing method, including (*a*) inability to measure and control temperature, environmental pollutants, or allergens; (*b*) inability to measure and control work; and (*c*) inability to monitor EKG, oxygen saturation, and blood pressure.

Table 4.1: Severity of EIA according to percent fall in PEFR or FEV$_1$ from the preexercise level

Severity	% Fall
Mild	10–25
Moderate	25–35
Moderate/Severe	35–50
Severe	>50

The treadmill should be set with little or no grade and slow speed to start. In adults, the grade and speed should be increased in several steps during the first 4 minutes to allow careful observation of EKG, SaO$_2$, and blood pressure.

A target heart rate of 80 to 90% of the patient's maximum heart rate (approximately 220 − age) should be achieved by the fourth minute of exercise. After reaching the target heart rate, an additional 4 to 6 minutes of steady-state (constant workload) exercise should be maintained.

Noseclips should be worn to ensure mouth breathing. If possible, the ambient temperature and humidity should be measured and noted on the report.

PFTs should be measured prior to exercise and approximately 5 minutes after exercise ends. If EIA is not apparent, PFTs should be measured again approximately 15 to 20 minutes after exercise ends.

If EIA is documented by PFTs, inhaled bronchodilators should be administered. Further EIA testing is not required. The laboratory may want to remeasure PFTs after bronchodilator to ensure that the patient has recovered before leaving. Occasionally, the EIA is so severe that PFTs cannot be obtained and treatment is required immediately. This should be documented in the report, and postbronchodilator PFTs should be performed before the patient leaves.

The importance of the inspired air temperature and humidity has been discussed. It may be necessary to have some patients breathe cold, dry air during the exercise period. A commercially available heat exchanger (Turboaire Challenger, Equilibrated Bio Systems, Inc., Melville, New York), which requires a compressed air source, will deliver very cold, dry air to the mouth. In my experience, cold, dry air may be necessary with the occasional patient who does not have a large enough fall in ventilatory function when breathing air at room temperature and humidity.

When the purpose of the EIA test is to evaluate pharmacotherapy, the drug or drugs being evaluated should be administered in time to take effect

Table 4.2: Spirometry on a 20-year-old asthmatic man before and after two puffs of albuterol from a metered dose inhaler

	Before RX	After RX
FVC (L)	5.24 (87)*	5.49
FEV$_1$ (L)	3.80 (79)	4.56
FEV$_1$/FVC (%)	73	83
FEF25-75 (L/sec)	2.59 (45)	3.48

*Values in parentheses are percent of predicted

Table 4.3: Spirometry on a 20-year-old asthmatic man before and after treadmill exercise

	Before	5' After	20' After
FVC (L)	5.33	5.29	5.30
FEV$_1$ (L)	3.99	3.83	3.85
FEV$_1$/FVC (%)	75	72	73
FEF25-75% (L/sec)	2.78	2.61	2.62

prior to exercise. Pulmonary function tests should then be obtained and exercise performed in the manner described.

CASE 4.1

A 20-year-old man was admitted to the hospital because of increasing problems with his asthma. The major complaint was that his asthma attacks were restricting his sports activities, especially in the winter months. He enjoyed basketball, soccer, and cycling but had adopted a sedentary lifestyle because of increased problems with asthma. He often pretreated himself with aerosolized bronchodilators before exercise but claimed that such pretreatment had not been effective.

His admission spirometry is shown in Table 4.2. These results are consistent with airflow limitation, with good response to bronchodilator.

The next day, spirometry was done before and after treadmill exercise, and the results are shown in Table 4.3. These results suggest the patient *does not* have exercise-induced asthma.

The bronchospastic response to exercise is accentuated when asthmatics breathe cold, dry air (compared to the response when they breathe air at standard room conditions).[6,7,21] Strauss further notes that environmental conditions influence the magnitude of response.[7] Thus, variations in environmental temperature and humidity are significant interactive variables that must be controlled.

The patient was rescheduled for treadmill exercise breathing cold, dry air. The speed, grade, and exercise time were kept close to those used in the first

Table 4.4: Spirometry on a 20-year-old asthmatic man before and after treadmill exercise breathing cold, dry air

	Before	5' After	% Change
FVC (L)	5.29	4.51	−15
FEV$_1$ (L)	3.89	2.93	−25
FEV$_1$/FVC (%)	74	65	
FEF25-75 (L/sec)	2.61	1.82	−30

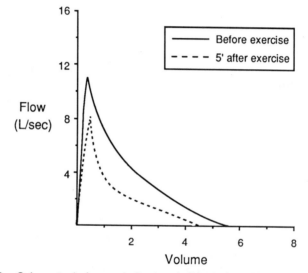

Figure 4.3. Spirometry before and after treadmill exercise while breathing cold, dry air.

Table 4.5: Spirometry on a 20-year-old asthmatic man before and after pretreatment and treadmill exercise while breathing cold, dry air

	Before RX	After RX	5' After Ex	20' After Ex
FVC (L)	5.21	5.37	5.29	5.31
FEV$_1$ (L)	3.79	4.49	4.27	4.29
FEV$_1$/FVC (%)	73	84	81	81
FEF25-75 (L/sec)	2.41	3.29	3.13	3.20

test. The results (shown in Table 4.4 and Figure 4.3) clearly demonstrate exercise-induced asthma.

The issue of appropriate pretreatment was addressed on a third exercise day. The patient was again exercised on the treadmill, breathing cold, dry air, but after pretreatment with albuterol (two puffs from a metered dose inhaler) and cromolyn sodium (two puffs from a metered dose inhaler). The results (shown in Table 4.5) reveal the effectiveness of this pretreatment.

Despite a positive history this patient did not demonstrate exercise-induced asthma in the laboratory until cold, dry air was added. Additionally, medication was shown to be effective in blocking the reaction to exercise and thus will be helpful in the management of this patient.

EXERCISE TOLERANCE TEST

The exercise tolerance test (sometimes called the "complete" exercise test) is the most useful test to determine the causes of dyspnea on exertion. In addition to its usefulness in making a differential diagnosis, it can also be used to determine disease severity and to evaluate the effects of therapy.

The procedure, which usually includes arterial blood gases, expired gas collection and analysis, EKG, and blood pressure, has become increasingly popular over the last 10 years. This is due, in part, to the numerous articles that were published in the 1960s and 1970s describing its usefulness and to technologic advances that have improved some of the older methods. Additionally, the exercise tolerance test is being used to evaluate the effectiveness of pulmonary rehabilitation procedures.

This section will discuss the exercise tolerance test and focus on the physiologic responses to exercise, instrumentation, techniques, protocols, calculations, and the basic elements of interpretation.

Physiology

The transition from rest to exercise requires the interaction of many physiologic and biochemical mechanisms. To discuss all of them would require an entire chapter, if not an entire book. However, the responses to exercise can be grouped into two broad categories: (*a*) **pulmonary responses** and (*b*) **cardiovascular responses** (including gas exchange responses).

The most basic pulmonary response to exercise is an increase in ventilation. The measurement of the increase in ventilation is usually made by measuring the volume of exhaled air and reporting it as the expired ventilation per minute ($\dot{V}E$). The $\dot{V}E$ consists of the alveolar ventilation per minute ($\dot{V}A$) and dead space ventilation per minute ($\dot{V}D$), that is, $\dot{V}E = \dot{V}A + \dot{V}D$. The respiratory rate (f) and tidal volume (VT) are also reported.

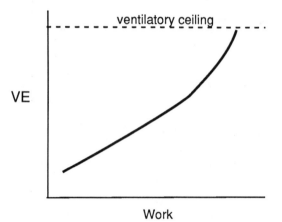

Figure 4.4. Normal ventilatory response to increasing exercise is linear up to the point when metabolism becomes anaerobic, after which it increases faster.

Ventilation increases with exercise. At low and moderate levels of exercise, ventilation increases in a linear manner up to approximately 50% of maximum $\dot{V}O_2$. At higher levels of exercise, ventilation increases relatively more, up to the "ventilatory ceiling" (Figure 4.4). This ceiling is the maximum volume one can achieve during exertion. It can be approximated by measuring the volume one can generate performing a maximal voluntary ventilation test (MVV), which has the patient breathe in and out as deep and as fast as possible for 10 to 15 seconds. The total amount of air breathed out during that short period is then extrapolated to liters per minute. An alternative to the MVV test is to estimate the ceiling by multiplying the FEV_1 by 35 or 41.[3,22] During exercise, one cannot maintain his/her MVV or ceiling for long periods. In fact, at a healthy individual's maximum $\dot{V}O_2$, ventilation is only approximately 60 to 70% of the MVV.[23]

The increase in ventilation is achieved first by increases in tidal volume (VT). However, the size of the tidal breaths is limited, and, at approximately 60% of the vital capacity, VT increases level off and frequency increases. Figure 4.5 shows the relationships of frequency and tidal volume to ventilation.

As work increases, the exercising muscles demand more oxygen (O_2) and must eliminate more carbon dioxide (CO_2). The relationship among $\dot{V}O_2$, work, and ventilation is linear. At the point at which anaerobic metabolism begins, ventilation increases faster than $\dot{V}O_2$ and work. As a result, arterial CO_2 tension ($PaCO_2$) remains fairly constant in healthy individuals until anaerobic metabolism begins, and then it begins to fall. These relationships are shown in Figures 4.6 and 4.7.

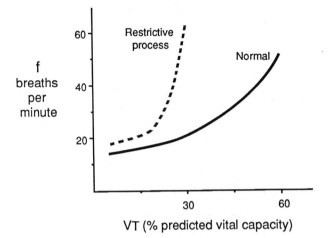

Figure 4.5. Increases in ventilation due to exercise are accomplished by increases in tidal volume (VT) and respiratory frequency (f). In normal individuals, the increases in ventilation are primarily achieved by increases in VT. However, at high levels of exercise, f plays more of a role. VT increases up to approximately 60% of the patient's vital capacity and levels off, while f increases up to 50 to 60 breaths per minute. If the relationship between f and VT is shifted upward and to the left (*dashed line*), more rapid and shallow breathing occurs, which is commonly seen in patients with restrictive processes.

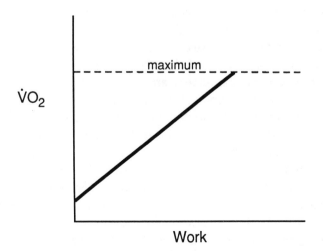

Figure 4.6. Oxygen consumption ($\dot{V}O_2$) increases linearly with work.

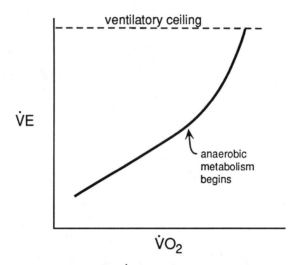

Figure 4.7. Oxygen consumption ($\dot{V}O_2$) increases linearly with ventilation up to an-aerobic metabolism, at which point ventilation increases faster than $\dot{V}O_2$.

With each tidal breath, part of the inspired air reaches the alveoli and part remains in the conducting airways. The gas in the conducting airways and respiratory units that are not perfused do not take part in gas exchange and are referred to as **dead space** (VD). Dead space includes the con-ducting airways and mainstream bronchi (anatomic dead space), as well as those respiratory units that are not perfused (physiologic dead space). Nor-mally, at rest, the VD is approximately 30% of the VT. For example, if the VT is 700 ml, the amount of anatomic and physiologic dead space is approxi-mately 210 ml. During exercise, this ratio of VD to VT normally falls to between 5 and 25% as the result of the increase in VT.

In order to increase blood flow to the exercising muscles, **the body's main cardiovascular response is an increase in cardiac output.** The cardiac output is the amount of blood pumped by each ventricle per min-ute and is the product of stroke volume and heart rate. Initially, both the stroke volume and heart rate increase but the relative increases depend on the nature of the exercise and on the physical condition of the individual. However, when the heart rate reaches approximately 110 to 130 beats/min, the rate of increase by stroke volume diminishes. The relationship of heart rate to oxygen consumption is linear within an individual and is shown in Figure 4.8.

Systemic blood pressure also increases during exercise in healthy indi-viduals. The increase in systolic blood pressure at maximal exercise is gen-

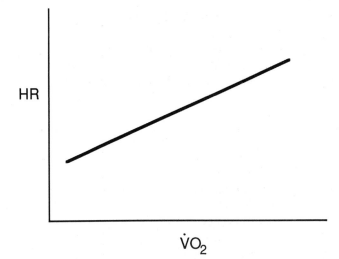

Figure 4.8. The relationship of heart rate (HR) to oxygen consumption ($\dot{V}O_2$) is linear within an individual.

erally 80 to 150 mm Hg above the resting level. The diastolic blood pressure rises very little and generally remains near resting levels.

The concept of **anaerobic threshold** is used by many to describe the onset of oxygen debt in exercising muscle—in other words, it is the level at which muscle metabolism switches from an anaerobic process because of an inadequate supply of oxygen. Consequently, the lactic acid concentration in the blood and the $\dot{V}CO_2$ rise abruptly. The $\dot{V}CO_2$ increase results from the increased reactions of lactic acid and bicarbonate. The changes in these easily measured parameters allow easy identification of the anaerobic threshold. However, its usefulness is questionable, and its determination is not an exact science.

Protocols

Many different exercise protocols can be used to evaluate a patient's exercise tolerance. For simplicity I will present two main types: (*a*) a **symptom-limited maximum protocol** and (*b*) a **constant-work steady-state protocol**.

The **symptom-limited maximal exercise protocol**, probably the most commonly used method, starts with a low workload that is increased incrementally (in equal or unequal amounts) so that the patient reaches a maximum exertion level (exhaustion) within 7 to 12 minutes. The workload is increased every 1 to 3 minutes, but caution should be used so that the patient does not become prematurely fatigued.

The **steady-state exercise protocol** is based on the fact that an individual can be exercised at a fixed submaximal workload for a long period of time without exhaustion. The submaximal workload permits the ventilatory and cardiovascular responses to become adapted to this exercise level and remain constant from minute to minute. Generally, it takes about 3 minutes for this equilibration to occur, and measurements are taken between the fourth and sixth minutes.

Both protocols are useful. The maximal exercise protocol, which requires the patient to work harder and harder until exhaustion, is used to determine the workload at which maximum oxygen consumption occurs. It is the preferred protocol when it is desirable to evaluate the extent of any limitation and the factors contributing to it and to see what other symptoms may appear.

The steady-state protocol, which uses a constant workload, allows for precise measurements at a given oxygen consumption level. However, I think this protocol's real value is in the fact that a patient can be exercised at various points in time (e.g., every 6 months; before and after therapy) at the same steady state workload. Then, comparisons can be made of the many parameters (e.g., $\dot{V}O_2$, VD/VT, PaO_2, etc.) to evaluate changes.

Instrumentation

The **treadmill** and **cycle ergometer** are devices used to exercise the patient, with the **treadmill** being the more commonly used of the two. The treadmill allows walking and/or running—activities that are familiar to both the old and the young patient. The treadmill has also been shown to produce a slightly higher maximum O_2 consumption. However, the treadmill is big, heavy, noisy, and potentially dangerous if the patient should fall.

The **cycle ergometer**, which is becoming more and more popular, is the more practical device in my opinion. It is smaller and quieter, can be moved from room to room, allows for easier blood pressure measurements and arterial blood sampling, and is safer in terms of the patient falling. Additionally, the electronically braked cycle maintains the workload even if the patient reduces the pedaling speed.

The **electrocardiograph** should be capable of performing a 12-lead measurement with minimal motion artifact. Most devices available at time of writing (1991) are capable of filtering "noise" caused by motion, thus allowing better monitoring capabilities.

A manual **blood pressure** measuring device (sphygmomanometer) is necessary and should be available even if the laboratory uses an automatic blood pressure measuring device or measures blood pressure directly from the arterial line via pressure transducer.

The **pulse oximeter** should be used as a monitor. The operation and pitfalls of using this device are discussed in detail in the section on exercise for desaturation with oximetry.

The measurement of oxygen consumption, carbon dioxide production, and minute ventilation requires several components. In the past a patient would breathe on a one-direction valve and the exhaled gas was collected in large (e.g., 120-liter) Tissot spirometer or meteorologic balloon. A small sample of this exhaled gas would be drawn off and analyzed on a gas chromatograph or Scholander manometric device. This cumbersome process took many hours and several technicians.

Today, minute ventilation is generally measured by electronically integrating the flow signal obtained by using a pneumotach, hot-wire anemometer, or turbine. The commercial systems generally measure exhaled flow and report exhaled volume. In my laboratory, we have put together a system that measures both inspiratory and expiratory flows and thus measures inspired and expired volumes.

Oxygen is analyzed using the paramagnetic, polarographic, zirconia cell, or mass spectrometry principles. The paramagnetic and polarographic analyzers are widely used in respiratory care and are small, inexpensive, and relatively slow in response. The zirconia cell analyzer is much faster in response than the paramagnetic and polarographic analyzers but requires extremely high temperature to operate. Although the mass spectrometer is the fastest analyzer, it is also the largest and most expensive. At the time of writing (1991), most commercial exercise systems available use the zirconium analyzer.

Carbon dioxide is analyzed by the infrared analyzer or mass spectrometer. The infrared analyzer is the slower of the two but is smaller, much less expensive, and used in most commercial exercise systems.

These gas analyzers and computer technology have greatly reduced the total time required for analysis and computations and the number of technicians.

Computerization has enabled these systems, sometimes referred to as "metabolic carts," to sample data frequently and to average results. Data

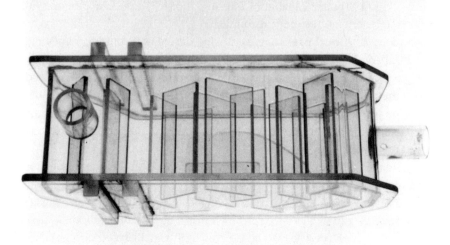

Figure 4.9. A mixing chamber with inlet, outlet, and a series of baffles to mix the exhaled gas. (Photograph by Barry Silverstein.)

sampling is accomplished using one of two systems: (*a*) **breath by breath** or (*b*) **mixing chamber.**

The **breath-by-breath** systems measure data continuously during each breath. Thus ventilation, O_2 consumption, and CO_2 production are measured during each breath and then totaled over a given time period. The gas analyzers must be rapid, and response times of both the analyzers and the volume measuring device must be synchronized. The advantage of the breath-by-breath method is the ability to measure all the values rapidly, thus enabling the workload to be increased sooner and more data points to be collected.

The **mixing chamber** systems use a small chamber (2 to 6 liters) on the exhaled side of the one-way valve. As the exhaled gas enters the chamber, it travels through and is mixed by a series of baffles or struts as shown in Figure 4.9. The gas becomes homogeneous and exits at the outlet of the chamber, where it is sampled and analyzed by the O_2 and CO_2 analyzers. This method does not require the high-speed O_2 analyzers and the adjustment for time delays as in the breath-by-breath method.

The breathing valves are often used to separate inspired from expired gas. The valves shown in Figure 4.10 are commonly used types. These valves must have low resistance and low dead space and be easy to clean. Some vendors have eliminated the valve and use a flow-

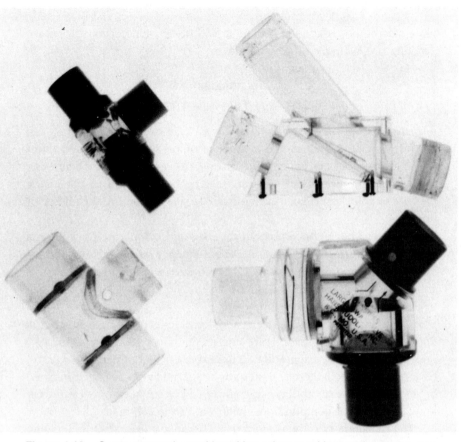

Figure 4.10. Some commonly used breathing valves used in exercise-testing systems. (Photograph by Barry Silverstein.)

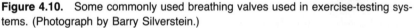

measuring device such as a pneumotach at the patient's mouth. The advantage of replacing the valve is that resistance is eliminated and the dead space is reduced. However, cleaning is not always easy. Additionally, patients who require increased inspired oxygen concentrations when they exercise need a one-way valve to separate the inspired and expired gases.

Patient Preparation

In almost all cases, it is not necessary to withhold medications. In fact, there may be an effort to ensure that a patient has taken all prescribed medications.

Because EKG leads must be applied and because arterial blood sampling may be necessary, the patient should dress appropriately. Shoes for pedaling or walking should also be worn.

Techniques

ARTERIAL LINE INSERTION

In many laboratories, arterial blood gas samples are obtained at rest and during exercise. However, the number of blood samples obtained varies from laboratory to laboratory, and in some cases samples are obtained as often as every minute during exercise. The best method to obtain numerous samples, especially during exercise, is via an arterial catheter or line.

There has been concern about the risks and complications of arterial line insertion (arterial cannulation). The frequency of major complications from arterial line insertion is small,[24] infections related to arterial catheters are low,[25] and ultrasound and Allen's test application disclose a low incidence of radial artery occlusion.[26]

There also has been a concern about problems resulting from arterial line insertion by respiratory care and/or pulmonary function laboratory personnel. In my experience and in the experience of others with whom I have communicated, literally thousands of arterial lines have been inserted by respiratory care and pulmonary function laboratory personnel with very low rates of major complications, infection, or thrombosis.

The radial artery is the preferred site because it is accessible, and adequate collateral circulation is usually present and easily checked. The brachial artery should be used only if the radial sites are unavailable or attempts have been unsuccessful.

The two methods of inserting a catheter into an artery are (*a*) **transfixing the artery** (that is, deliberately puncturing the posterior wall of the artery) and (*b*) **direct threading**, in which the posterior wall is not punctured. No significant difference in the incidence of thrombosis or serious complications exists between the two methods,[27] and the choice of one or the other is arbitrary. I prefer to use the direct threading technique.

Two methods are used to keep the arterial catheter "open" and free of clots. The first is the continuous flow technique using a pressure bag, transfer pack with heparinized solution, intravenous tubing, intraflo device, stopcocks, and tubing. A pressure transducer can also be incorporated to measure arterial blood pressure. The second method is the noncontinuous technique, which requires the injection of a small amount of heparinized saline into the catheter and tubing after each blood sample has been withdrawn.

Prior to inserting the catheter, choose the site and perform the modified Allen's test, which requires the ulnar artery to fill the empty capillary beds in the hand within 10 to 15 seconds. Next, prepare the site by positioning the arm so that the wrist is slightly hyperextended and the palm is facing up. A rolled towel under the wrist may facilitate the positioning. Cleanse the skin at the puncture site with a betadine solution, followed by an alcohol swab.

Wear rubber or latex gloves while inserting the catheter to avoid possible contact with the blood.

Use a small-gauge needle (e.g., 25 gauge) to inject, subcutaneously around the site, a small amount (1 to 3 ml) of 1 or 2% lidocaine anesthetic (without epinephrine) if the patient is not allergic. Be careful not to inject into the artery. The raised skin bleb created when the anesthetic is injected will diminish within 1 to 5 minutes.

Wait for the anesthetic to become effective (5 to 10 minutes), and identify the position of the artery with the second and third fingers. In using the direct threading technique, one should insert the heparinized catheter into the skin at approximately a 30-degree angle with the bevel facing up. Advance until a "flash" (blood filling the hub) is obtained, then advance approximately one more millimeter to ensure that the needle and catheter are both in the artery. Slowly advance the catheter into the artery as you withdraw the needle. The catheter should advance smoothly. Do not try to force it. If the needle does not advance smoothly, the catheter is not in the artery lumen and withdrawal may be necessary. If the catheter must be withdrawn, hold pressure with sterile gauze for 3 to 5 minutes.

The properly inserted catheter will eject arterial blood in a pulsating manner. Therefore, it is a good idea to insert it with a stopcock and tubing attached or within easy reach so blood does not squirt all over you and your patient. The properly inserted catheter should then be taped to prevent inadvertent removal. I recommend that a thin strip of tape be looped around the hub and attached to the wrist. A second strip should be placed over the hub and onto the skin. A piece of sterile gauze can also be placed under the hub prior to taping. Armboards are useful and remind everyone involved that there is a catheter in the arm.

Flush the catheter with the heparinized solution to ensure that it remains patent. Before withdrawing any arterial blood samples for analysis, withdraw and discard a small amount (1 to 3 ml depending on the length of the tubing) of solution (blood and saline mixture) so that the sample will be pure.

REST MEASUREMENTS

The measurement of resting physiologic parameters is relatively simple compared to measurement during exercise. However, there still are some important points to remember.

The patient must be in a steady state. The wearing of noseclips, breathing on a mouthpiece and valve, having an arterial line, technicians and doctor moving around and talking, and other distractions can take some getting used to. However, 4 or 5 minutes of quiet breathing on the mouthpiece in the sitting position are usually adequate for equilibration, after which the physiologic data can be collected. In my experience 2 or 3 minutes of collection usually provide a good baseline assessment. If the resting data from a computerized system are immediately available they should be reviewed to ensure reproducibility and reasonability. The EKG and blood pressure at rest should also be examined to ensure that they do not contraindicate exercise.

The blood gas data should also be examined for reasonability and for hypoxemia. It is common to have patients who have a resting oxyhemoglobin saturation of <90%. In these cases, rest and exercise tests may be desired on both room air and supplemental oxygen.

For tests on increased levels of oxygen, remember that the FIO_2 must remain constant. A simple and inexpensive approach is to fill a large reservoir bag with the desired gas mixture and attach it to the inspired side of the one-way valve. Compressed gas cylinders with various O_2 concentrations can be kept on hand, or a blender can be employed to keep the bag filled.

EXERCISE MEASUREMENTS

After satisfactory resting data have been obtained, the patient can remain on the mouthpiece and go directly into the exercise protocol. However, another approach that works better in some cases is to allow the patient to come off the mouthpiece for a short period. Frequently, he/she may need to cough or swallow. Exercise directions can also be given or repeated at this time—immediately before the exercise period.

As mentioned earlier, there are two major exercise protocol strategies: (*a*) a steady-state protocol and (*b*) a symptom-limited maximum protocol. In a steady-state protocol, one workload is used for a specific period of time (e.g., 6 minutes). However, if maximum oxygen consumption is desired, the symptom-limited maximum protocol must be used, in which the workload is initially low and increased at intervals until the patient is exhausted.

The best-known and most commonly used treadmill protocols are the Bruce and Balke protocols,[28,29] which have been modified in some published articles.[30-32]

The cycle ergometer protocol developed by Jones and colleagues[33] (one of several) starts the exercise at 16 watts and increases the work level 16 watts every minute. One variation of this protocol, which starts the exercise at 8 watts, is frequently used in unfit and dyspneic patients. My experience has been that many patients entering a pulmonary rehabilitation program have difficulty starting much above 5 watts, and therefore some variation may be needed.

CALCULATIONS

Although most laboratories are equipped with computers that calculate all or some of the reported parameters, the student and practitioner can better understand how the data are analyzed by studying more commonly used formulas and related information.

Minute ventilation ($\dot{V}E$) is the volume of air a patient exhales in one minute expressed in liters per minute, at body temperature and pressure saturated with water vapor (BTPS). The **tidal volume** (VT) is also reported in BTPS and calculated as follows:

$$\text{VT (liters at BTPS)} = \frac{\dot{V}E \text{ (liters per minute at BTPS)}}{\text{respiratory frequency per minute}}$$

Oxygen consumption ($\dot{V}O_2$) is the amount of oxygen consumed by the body each minute. It is calculated from the minute ventilation at standard temperature and pressure dry (STPD) and the difference between the inspired and expired oxygen concentrations. The calculation of $\dot{V}O_2$ is complicated by a correction for nitrogen and water vapor. But in its simplest form, $\dot{V}O_2$ can be calculated as follows:

$$\dot{V}O_2 \text{ (liters per minute at STPD)} = (FIO_2 \times \dot{V}I_{STPD}) - (FEO_2 \times \dot{V}E_{STPD})$$

Where: FIO_2 is the fractional concentration of dry oxygen inspired; FEO_2 is the fractional concentration of dry oxygen exhaled; $\dot{V}I_{STPD}$ is the volume of inspired air per minute at STPD; $\dot{V}E_{STPD}$ is the volume of exhaled air per minute at STPD.

The conversion of volumes from ambient conditions to standard conditions (STPD) is described in the appendix.

Carbon dioxide production ($\dot{V}CO_2$) is the amount of CO_2 produced by the body each minute. It is calculated from the minute ventilation at STPD and the difference between the inspired and expired CO_2 concentrations. The formula for calculating $\dot{V}CO_2$ is as follows:

$$\dot{V}CO_2 \text{ (liters per minute at STPD)} = \dot{V}E_{STPD} \times (FECO_2 - FICO_2)$$

Where: $\dot{V}E_{STPD}$ is the volume of exhaled air per minute at STPD; $FECO_2$ is the fractional concentration of dry exhaled CO_2; $FICO_2$ is the fractional concentration of dry inhaled CO_2 (usually 0.04%).

The **respiratory quotient** or **gas exchange ratio** (R) measures the relationship of carbon dioxide production to oxygen consumption and is calculated as follows:

$$R = \frac{\dot{V}CO_2}{\dot{V}O_2}$$

Oxygen pulse ($\dot{V}O_2/HR$) is a measurement that determines the amount of oxygen consumption per heartbeat and is calculated as follows:

$$\dot{V}O_2/HR = \frac{\dot{V}O_2 \times 1000}{HR}$$

Where: $\dot{V}O_2$ is oxygen consumption in ml per minute; HR is heart rate in beats per minute; 1000 is conversion from liters to ml.

The **ventilatory equivalent for O_2** ($\dot{V}E/\dot{V}O_2$) measures the ventilation requirement for a given oxygen consumption. Likewise the **ventilatory equivalent for CO_2** ($\dot{V}E/\dot{V}CO_2$) measures the ventilation requirement for a given amount of carbon dioxide production. These two measurements are calculated as follows:

$$\dot{V}E/\dot{V}O_2 = \frac{\dot{V}E - (f \times VDM)}{\dot{V}O_2} \text{ and,}$$

$$\dot{V}E/\dot{V}CO_2 = \frac{\dot{V}E - (f \times VDM)}{\dot{V}CO_2}$$

Where: $\dot{V}E/\dot{V}O_2$ is O_2 ventilatory equivalent; $\dot{V}E/\dot{V}CO_2$ is CO_2 ventilatory equivalent; $\dot{V}E$ is volume of exhaled air at BTPS in liters per minute; f is respiratory frequency per minute; VDM is valve dead space per breath in liters; $\dot{V}O_2$ is oxygen consumption at STPD in liters per minute; $\dot{V}CO_2$ is carbon dioxide production at STPD in liters per minute.

The **physiologic dead space** (VD) is the portion of each tidal breath that does not take part in gas exchange. It includes the volume of the anatomic dead space and those respiratory units that are ventilated but not perfused. The calculation of VD is as follows

$$VD = VT \times \frac{PaCO_2 - PECO_2}{PaCO_2} - VDM$$

Where: VD is physiologic dead space in liters; VT is tidal volume in liters at BTPS; $PaCO_2$ is arterial carbon dioxide tension in mm Hg; $PECO_2$ is mixed expired carbon dioxide concentration in mm Hg; VDM is valve dead space.

The ratio of the physiologic dead space volume to tidal breath volume (**VD/VT**) is calculated as follows:

$$VD/VT = \frac{VD}{VT}$$

Where: VD is physiologic dead space in liters; VT is tidal volume in liters.

The use of these complex equations is best illustrated by the following example of a healthy man. The exercise test was conducted on a cycle ergometer with a constant workload of 120 watts for 6 minutes. The following information is given: minute ventilation ($\dot{V}E$) at BTPS = 75 liters/min; minute ventilation ($\dot{V}E$) at STPD = 54 liters/min; respiratory frequency (f) = 35 breaths/min; assume $\dot{V}I = \dot{V}E$; inspired oxygen concentration (FIO_2) = 0.2093; expired oxygen concentration (FEO_2) = 0.1650; inspired carbon dioxide concentration ($FICO_2$) = 0.0004; expired carbon dioxide concentration ($FECO_2$) = 0.0450; heart rate (HR) = 150 beats/min; valve dead space (VDM) = 0.040 liters; arterial blood carbon dioxide tension ($PaCO_2$) = 35 mm Hg; mixed expired carbon dioxide tension ($PECO_2$) = 29 mm Hg.

Calculate the following parameters:

VT, $\dot{V}O_2$, $\dot{V}CO_2$, R, O_2 pulse, ventilatory equivalent for O_2 and CO_2, VD, and VD/VT.

1. $VT = \dfrac{\dot{V}E}{f} = \dfrac{75 \text{ liters/min}}{35} = 2.14 \text{ liters}$

2. $\dot{V}O_2 = (FIO_2 \times VI_{STPD}) - (FEO_2 \times \dot{V}E_{STPD}) = 0.2093\,(54) - 0.1650\,(54)$

  $\dot{V}O_2 = 11.30 - 8.91 = 2.39 \text{ liters/min}$

3. $\dot{V}CO_2 = \dot{V}E_{STPD} \times (FECO_2 - FICO_2)$
   $= 54 \times (0.0450 - 0.0004)$
   $= 2.41 \text{ liters/min}$

4. $R = \dfrac{\dot{V}CO_2}{\dot{V}O_2} = \dfrac{2.41}{2.39} = 1.01$

5. $O_2 \text{ pulse} = \dfrac{\dot{V}O_2 \times 1000}{HR} = \dfrac{2.39 \times 1000}{150} = 15.93$

6. O_2 ventilatory equivalent

$$\dot{V}E/\dot{V}O_2 = \dfrac{\dot{V}E - (f \times VDM)}{\dot{V}O_2} = \dfrac{75 - (35 \times 0.040)}{2.39} = 30.8$$

7. CO_2 ventilatory equivalent

$$\dot{V}E/\dot{V}CO_2 = \dfrac{\dot{V}E - (f \times VDM)}{\dot{V}CO_2} = \dfrac{75 - (35 \times 0.040)}{2.41} = 30.5$$

8. $VD = VT \times \dfrac{PaCO_2 - PECO_2}{PaCO_2} - VDM$

$$= 2.14 \times \dfrac{35 - 29}{35} = 0.327 \text{ liters}$$

9. $VD/VT = \dfrac{VD}{VT} = \dfrac{0.327}{2.14} = 0.153$

Case Presentations and Basic Elements of Interpretation

The basic elements of interpretation are presented through a series of cases. Each case briefly describes the patient and the exercise protocol. Each case also displays a table of rest and exercise data and two panels of four graphs each. The data in the tables are limited and more graphs could be presented, but I have elected to keep things simple and concise.

CASE 4.2

A healthy 21-year-old local college cross-country runner was tested in the pulmonary function laboratory. He complained of having had a recent series of viral upper respiratory infections that were causing a "lung problem" that was affecting his running. His coach was concerned about his recent level of dyspnea and

Table 4.6: Ventilatory, cardiovascular, and gas exchange measurements from the final minutes of rest and maximal exercise in Case 4.2

	Rest	Max Exercise
Workload (watts on cycle)	0	350 (95)*
$\dot{V}E$ (L/min)	13.8	170.8 (134)
$\dot{V}O_2$ (L/min)	0.300	4.20 (95)
$\dot{V}OC_2$ (L/min)	0.250	4.31
R	0.83	1.03
f (breaths/min)	14	40
VT (L)	0.986	4.270
VD (L)	0.291	1.110
VD/VT (%)	30	26
FIO_2	0.21	0.21
pH	7.43	7.31
$PaCO_2$ (torr)	35	32
PaO_2 (torr)	75$^\Delta$	74
HbO_2 (%)	95	95
$P(A-a)O_2$ (torr)	5.7	17.7
HR (beats/min)	68	193 (98)
Systolic blood pressure (torr)	118	161
Diastolic blood pressure (torr)	79	81

*Values in parentheses are percent of predicted maximum
$^\Delta$At 5000 feet, normal PaO_2s are approximately 65 to 75 torr

performance. His pulmonary function tests were normal with no improvement after bronchodilator.

A maximal, symptom-limited exercise test was ordered to determine whether a disease process was the cause of his dyspnea and poor performance.

An arterial catheter was placed in the radial artery to obtain blood gas samples. Twelve-lead EKG, blood pressure, minute ventilation, and expired gas concentrations were obtained. Resting parameters were obtained after the patient had breathed quietly on the mouthpiece for approximately 5 minutes. The exercise was performed on a cycle ergometer starting at 50 watts, with 50-watt increments every minute until exhaustion. The results of the rest and exercise test are shown in Table 4.6 and Figures 4.11 and 4.12.

Interpretation
Interpretation of exercise results is best approached by comparing the patient's rest and exercise response to a predicted response; however, the predicted values (as with all predicted or reference values) should be viewed as estimates or approximations.

The resting data in this patient show no abnormalities. The exercise response is broken into two sets of graph panels. The ventilatory response is displayed in Figure 4.11. The ventilatory response as measured by compar-

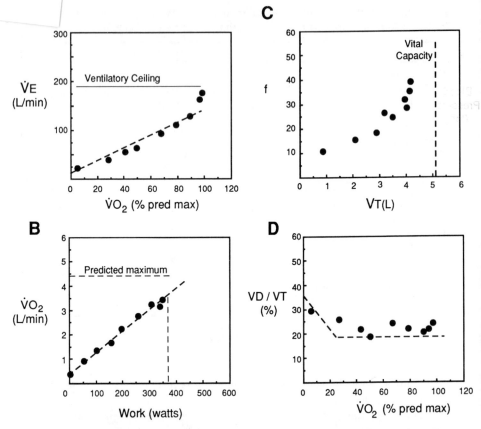

Figure 4.11. The ventilatory response of the 21-year-old man in Case 4.2. **A,** Expired minute ventilation ($\dot{V}E$) versus oxygen consumption ($\dot{V}O_2$, as a percent of predicted maximum), with predicted line (*dash*) and ventilatory ceiling calculated from $FEV_1 \times 40$. **B,** Workload versus oxygen consumption ($\dot{V}O_2$) with predicted line (*dash*). **C,** Respiratory rate (f) versus tidal volume (VT) with a vertical dashed line representing the patient's vital capacity. **D,** Dead space to tidal volume ratio (VD/VT) versus oxygen consumption ($\dot{V}O_2$, as percent of predicted maximum), with predicted response line (*dash*).

ing minute ventilation to O_2 consumption (Fig. 4.11*A*) is linear until about 90% of the maximum $\dot{V}O_2$ and then approaches the ventilatory ceiling. The relationship of $\dot{V}O_2$ to work rate is linear (i.e., increases in work should cause corresponding increases in $\dot{V}O_2$), and Figure 4.11*B* shows a normal response by this patient. The increase in ventilation was obtained by increasing the respiratory frequency and tidal volume until the higher workloads, when only increases in frequency were observed (Fig. 4.11*C*). The VD/VT ratio was

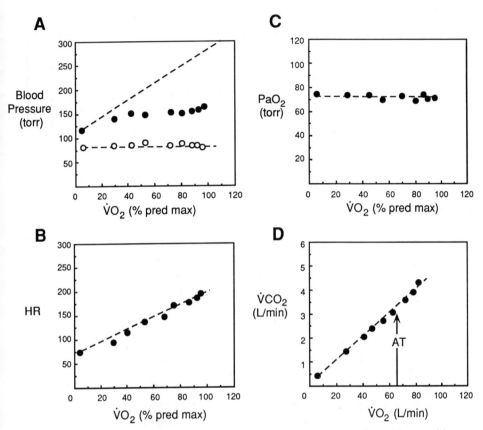

Figure 4.12. The cardiovascular and gas exchange responses of the 21-year-old man in Case 4.2. **A,** Systolic (●) and diastolic (O) blood pressure versus oxygen consumption ($\dot{V}O_2$, as a percent of predicted maximum) with normal response lines (*dash*). **B,** Heart rate (HR) versus oxygen consumption ($\dot{V}O_2$, as percent of predicted maximum) with normal response line (*dash*). **C,** PaO_2, versus oxygen consumption ($\dot{V}O_2$ as percent of predicted maximum) with normal response line (*dash*). **D,** Carbon dioxide production ($\dot{V}CO_2$) versus oxygen consumption ($\dot{V}O_2$) with normal response (*dashed line*) and anaerobic threshold point (AT).

30% at rest and fell to 26% at maximal exercise, and as Figure 4.11*D* shows, a normal response is a fall in the VD/VT ratio.

The second set of graphs (Fig. 4.12) shows the cardiovascular and gas exchange responses. The blood pressure response (Fig. 4.12*A*) is normal, with an increase in the systolic pressure and no change in the diastolic pressure. However, the systolic blood pressure did not increase much above 150 to 160 torr with increases in workload, although this could be within normal limits. The heart rate response is normal; the linear response is shown in Figure 4.12*B*. The

PaO_2 was normal at rest (altitude 5000 feet) and remained unchanged during exercise (Fig. 4.12C). The $P(A-a)O_2$ gradient in Table 4.6 was 5.7 at rest and increased to 17.7 at maximal exercise, a normal response.

The anaerobic threshold (AT), the point representing the failure of the acid-base buffering system to prevent metabolic acidosis, can be estimated in several ways. One method is to determine the inflection in the $\dot{V}CO_2$ versus $\dot{V}O_2$ graph (Fig. 4.12D) that corresponds to the increase in ventilation seen in Figure 4.9A. It occurs in this patient at approximately 70% of maximum $\dot{V}O_2$, which is appropriate for a fit runner.

There were no abnormalities in the EKG, and the overall impression is a normal exercise response with the possible exception of the systolic blood pressure. However, the fact that only 95% of the maximum predicted workload was achieved before the patient quit exercising is suspect in a well-trained athlete.

CASE 4.3

A 50-year-old man complaining of dyspnea was seen by the occupational medicine clinic as an outpatient. He had worked with beryllium for approximately 20 years and was a 40-pack-year smoker. His pulmonary function tests showed airflow limitation (FEV_1 = 2.33 liters or 61% predicted, and the FEV_1/FVC = 52%) with no improvement after bronchodilator and a reduced single breath carbon monoxide diffusing capacity (DLCO = 18.3 or 51% predicted, and DLCO/VA = 2.9 or 57% predicted). A maximal, symptom limited, multistage exercise test was ordered.

An arterial catheter was placed in the radial artery, a 12-lead EKG was applied, and resting data were obtained. The exercise was performed on a cycle ergometer starting at 20 watts with 30-watt increments each minute until exhaustion. The patient quit after approximately 6 minutes, complaining of leg fatigue, shortness of breath, and chest tightness. The results of the rest and exercise test are shown in Table 4.7 and Figures 4.13 and 4.14.

At rest, the data reveal a low PaO_2 and O_2 saturation (HbO_2) with a correspondingly widened alveolar-arterial O_2 gradient ($PA-aO_2$).

Figure 4.13A shows a normal linear ventilation response up to about 45% of maximum predicted $\dot{V}O_2$ and then an increase to the ventilatory ceiling. Oxygen consumption should increase linearly with work, and as Figure 4.13B shows, this patient's response was essentially linear; however he fell short of predicted maximums. The increases in ventilation were accomplished with appropriate recruitment of VT, but frequency was excessive at maximum exercise as shown in Figure 4.13C. The VD/VT was slightly elevated at rest and inappropriately increased during exercise as shown in Figure 4.13D.

The blood pressure response (Fig. 4.14A) shows a slight diastolic hypertensive response and a decreased systolic response. The heart rate response is excessive (Fig. 4.14B). The PaO_2 is low at rest and drops during exercise (Fig. 4.14C). The $A-aO_2$ gradient was elevated at rest and increased throughout exercise. Although widening of the $A-aO_2$ gradient is seen in healthy individuals, it is

Table 4.7: Ventilatory, cardiovascular, and gas exchange measurements from the final minutes of rest and maximal exercise in Case 4.3

	Rest	Max Exercise
Workload (watts on cycle)	0	170 (76)*
$\dot{V}E$ (L/min)	12.7	91.7 (105)
$\dot{V}O_2$ (L/min)	0.388	1.693 (60)
$\dot{V}CO_2$ (L/min)	0.298	1.928
R	0.77	1.14
f (breaths/min)	12	48
VT (L)	1.058	1.910
VD (L)	0.382	0.779
VD/VT (%)	36	41
FIO_2	0.21	0.21
pH	7.42	7.39
$PaCO_2$ (torr)	38	35
PaO_2 (torr)	52$^\Delta$	45
HbO_2 (%)	88	80
$P(A\text{-}a)O_2$	22	44
HR (beats/min)	78	167 (94)
Systolic blood pressure (torr)	124	150
Diastolic blood pressure (torr)	85	105

*Values in parentheses are percent of predicted maximum
$^\Delta$At 5000 feet normal PaO2 range is 65 to 75 torr

abnormally widened at rest in this patient and widens even more with exercise. The AT can be estimated from the inflection in the $\dot{V}CO_2$ versus $\dot{V}O_2$ graph (Fig. 4.14D). Although only an approximation, this point represents the failure of the acid-base buffering system to prevent metabolic acidosis and occurs in this patient at approximately 40 to 45% of maximum $\dot{V}O_2$, which is low.

No abnormalities were seen in the EKG, and the overall impression is that there was exercise limitation due to abnormal gas exchange and ventilatory abnormalities. Additionally, the cardiovascular response was excessive given the level of work achieved.

CASE 4.4

A 62-year-old woman was referred to the pulmonary rehabilitation program. She was a 90-pack-year smoker with an FEV_1 of 1.12 liters (44% predicted) and an FEV_1/FVC of 37%, with no response to bronchodilator. Her single breath carbon dioxide diffusing capacity (DLCO) was 12.7 ml/min/mm Hg (51% predicted). Prior to beginning the program a maximal, symptom-limited, multistage exercise test was performed.

An arterial catheter was placed in the radial artery, and a 12-lead EKG was applied. A room-air arterial blood sample revealed a PaO_2 of 53 torr and the HbO_2 was 88%. Thus it was decided to perform both the rest and exercise test-

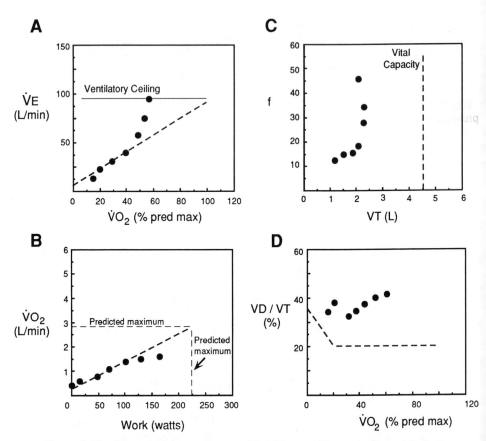

Figure 4.13.   The ventilatory response of the 50-year-old man in Case 4.3. **A,** Expired minute ventilation ($\dot{V}E$) versus oxygen consumption ($\dot{V}O_2$, as a percent of predicted maximum), with predicted line (*dash*) and ventilatory ceiling calculated from $FEV_1 \times 40$. **B,** Workload versus oxygen consumption ($\dot{V}O_2$) with predicted line (*dash*). **C,** Respiratory rate (f) versus tidal volume (VT) with a vertical dashed line representing the patient's vital capacity. **D,** Dead space to tidal volume ratio (VD/VT) versus oxygen consumption ($\dot{V}O_2$, as percent of predicted maximum), with predicted response line (*dash*).

ing with the patient breathing supplemental oxygen. A blender was used to produce 28% oxygen, which flowed to a large reservoir bag. The bag was connected to the inspired side of the one-way patient valve. The exercise was performed on a cycle ergometer starting at 5 watts and using 10-watt increments each minute until exhaustion. The patient quit after 6 minutes of exercise, complaining of shortness of breath and leg fatigue. The results of the exercise test are shown in Table 4.8 and Figures 4.15 and 4.16.

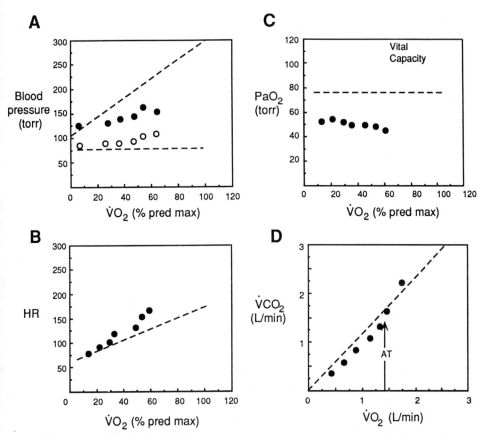

Figure 4.14. The cardiovascular and gas exchange responses of the 50-year-old man in Case 4.3. **A,** Systolic (●) and diastolic (○) blood pressure versus oxygen consumption ($\dot{V}O_2$, as a percent of predicted maximum) with normal response lines (*dash*). **B,** Heart rate (HR) versus oxygen consumption ($\dot{V}O_2$, as percent of predicted maximum) with normal response line (*dash*). **C,** PaO_2 versus oxygen consumption ($\dot{V}O_2$, as percent of predicted maximum) with normal response line (*dash*). **D,** Carbon dioxide production ($\dot{V}CO_2$) versus oxygen consumption ($\dot{V}O_2$) with normal response (*dashed line*) and anaerobic threshold point (AT).

Interpretation

The resting data reveal a low PaO_2 at rest on room air, which was normalized on supplemental oxygen (28%). The alveolar arterial oxygen gradient ($PA\text{-}aO_2$) is correspondingly widened, and the blood pressure is elevated.

The patient achieved a workload of 57% of the predicted maximum workload and a maximum $\dot{V}O_2$ that was 52% of predicted maximum.

Table 4.8: Ventilatory, cardiovascular, and gas exchange measurements from the final minutes of rest and maximal exercise in Case 4.4

	Test	Max Exercise
Workload (watts on cycle)	0	55 (57)*
$\dot{V}E$ (L/min)	14.3	42.0 (82)
$\dot{V}O_2$ (L/min)	0.316	0.707 (52)
$\dot{V}CO_2$ (L/min)	0.248	0.685
R	0.78	0.97
f (breaths/min)	14	27
VT (L)	1.021	1.556
VD (L)	0.379	0.709
VD/VT (%)	37	46
FIO_2	0.28	0.28
pH	7.41	7.34
$PaCO_2$ (torr)	30	31
PaO_2 (torr)	80	85
HbO_2 (%)	94	94
$P(A-aO_2)$	46	47
HR	96	141 (84)
Systolic blood pressure	175	249
Diastolic blood pressure	97	105

*Values in parentheses are percent of predicted maximum

Figure 4.15A shows that the minute ventilation increased excessively, reaching the ventilatory ceiling (which is low in this patient because of her airflow limitation) and probably limiting further exercise. Oxygen consumption increased linearly with work (a normal response), although only 52% of predicted maximum was achieved (Fig. 4.15B). The excessive increase in ventilation was accomplished mostly with excessive increases in respiratory rate (Fig. 4.15C). The VD/VT increased inappropriately during exercise (Fig. 4.15D).

Figure 4.16A shows the hypertensive response to exercise, although the heart rate response is normal (Fig. 4.16B). The alveolar arterial oxygen gradient $(PA-aO_2)$ was elevated at rest and remained elevated during exercise (Fig. 4.16C). No fall in the PaO_2 occurred with exercise. The AT approximation is seen at the inflection of the $\dot{V}CO_2$ and $\dot{V}O_2$ graph (Fig. 4.16D) and is approximately 45% of maximum, which is low.

No abnormalities in the EKG are seen, and the overall impression is that exercise limitation was due to ventilatory and cardiovascular abnormalities.

CASE 4.5

A 64-year-old man arrived in the pulmonary function laboratory for an exercise test. Pulmonary function tests on the previous day revealed:

Total lung capacity (TLC) = 58% predicted

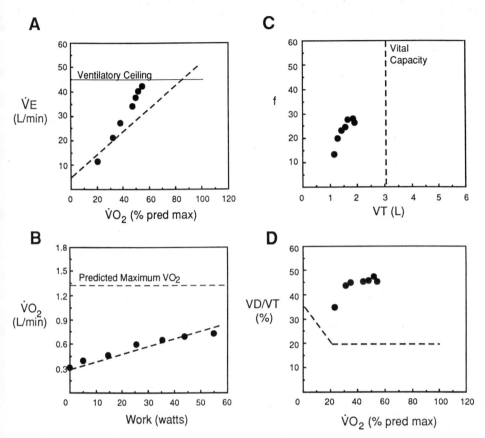

Figure 4.15. The ventilatory responses of the 62-year-old woman in Case 4.4. **A,** Expired minute ventilation ($\dot{V}E$) versus oxygen consumption ($\dot{V}O_2$, as a percent of predicted maximum), with predicted line (*dash*) and ventilatory ceiling calculated from $FEV_1 \times 40$. **B,** Workload versus oxygen consumption ($\dot{V}O_2$) with predicted line (*dash*). **C,** Respiratory rate (f) versus tidal volume (VT) with a vertical dashed line representing the patient's vital capacity. **D,** Dead space to tidal volume ratio (VD/VT) versus oxygen consumption ($\dot{V}O_2$, as percent of predicted maximum), with predicted response line (*dash*).

Forced vital capacity (FVC)	= 47% predicted
FEV_1/FVC	= 85%
Diffusing capacity (DLCO)	= 44% predicted
DLCO/VA	= 92% predicted

No response to bronchodilator was seen, and the patient claimed he had never smoked. These results are consistent with a restrictive process.

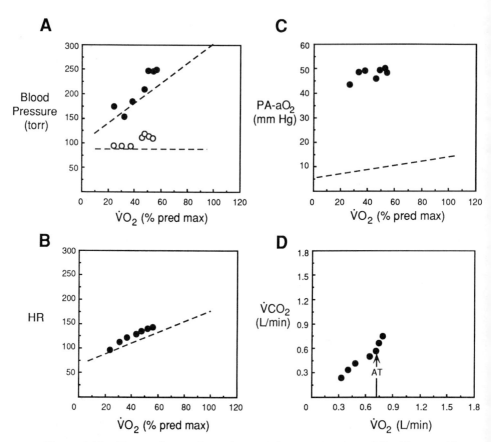

Figure 4.16. The cardiovascular and gas exchange responses of the 62-year-old woman in Case 4.4. **A,** Systolic (●) and diastolic (O) blood pressure versus oxygen consumption ($\dot{V}O_2$, as a percent of predicted maximum) with normal response lines (*dash*). **B,** Heart rate (HR) versus oxygen consumption ($\dot{V}O_2$, as percent of predicted maximum) with normal response line (*dash*). **C,** PA-aO_2 versus oxygen consumption ($\dot{V}O_2$, as percent of predicted maximum) with normal response line (*dash*). **D,** Carbon dioxide production ($\dot{V}CO_2$) versus oxygen consumption ($\dot{V}O_2$) with normal response (*dashed line*) and anaerobic threshold point (AT).

An arterial catheter was placed in the radial artery, and a 12-lead EKG was applied. Analysis of a room-air arterial blood sample revealed pH = 7.45, $PaCO_2$ = 35 mm Hg, PaO_2 = 60 mm Hg, SaO_2 = 90.5%. The PaO_2 is slightly low for 5000-feet altitude, but it was decided to exercise the patient on room air.

The exercise was performed on a cycle ergometer starting at 10 watts, and the workload was increased 10 watts every minute until exhaustion. The patient quit after 6 minutes of exercise despite hard coaching by the technicians. His

Table 4.9: Ventilatory, cardiovascular, and gas exchange measurements from the final minute of rest and maximal exercise in Case 4.5

	Rest	Max Exercise
Workload (watts on cycle)	0	60 (25)*
$\dot{V}E$ (L/min)	16.3	48.2 (55)
$\dot{V}O_2$ (L/min)	0.357	0.737 (24)
$\dot{V}CO_2$ (L/min)	0.296	0.578
R	0.83	0.78
f (breaths/min)	16	39
VT (L)	1.019	1.236
VD (L)	0.440	0.699
VD/VT (%)	43	57
FIO_2	0.21	0.21
pH	7.45	7.45
$PaCO_2$ (torr)	35	30
PaO_2 (torr)	60	55
HbO_2 (%)	91	89
$P(A-aO_2)$	19.6	27.8
HR	87	129
Systolic blood pressure (torr)	108	147
Diastolic blood pressure (torr)	68	93

*Values in parentheses are percent of predicted maximum

complaint was shortness of breath and dizziness. The results of this test are shown in Table 4.9 and Figures 4.17 and 4.18.

Interpretation
The resting data reveal a normal resting heart rate, slightly elevated minute ventilation, increased VD/VT, a slightly low PaO_2, and a widened alveolar-arterial oxygen gradient.

Figure 4.17*A* shows that minute ventilation is slightly high at rest and increases excessively for the level of oxygen consumption achieved. The ventilatory ceiling was not reached. The excessive increase in minute ventilation was achieved primarily with his increase in respiratory rate, with low tidal volumes remaining low (Fig. 4.17*C*). Oxygen consumption increased linearly with work (a normal response) up to approximately 30% of maximum $\dot{V}O_2$ (Fig. 4.17*B*). Additionally, only 58% of maximum $\dot{V}O_2$ was achieved. The VD/VT was increased at rest and inappropriately increased even more during exercise (Fig. 4.17*D*).

Figure 4.18*A* shows a normal resting blood pressure, but with exercise diastolic hypertension developed. The heart rate response (Fig. 4.18*B*) is excessive for the level of oxygen consumption achieved. The PaO_2 of 60 mm Hg breathing room air is slightly below the normal range at 5000-feet altitude. During exercise, the PaO_2 decreased slightly (Fig. 4.18*C*), which corresponds with the abnormal widening of the alveolar-arterial oxygen gradient. The pH remained unchanged during exercise, and

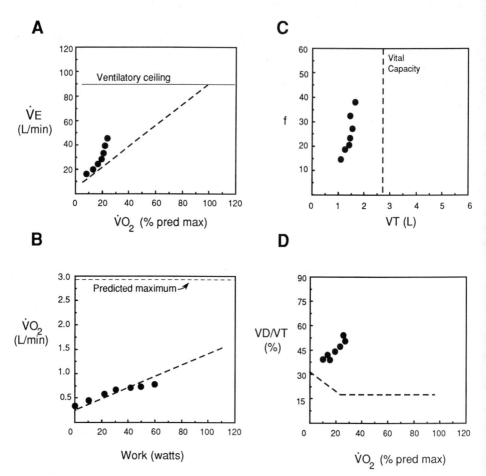

Figure 4.17. The ventilatory responses of the 64-year-old man in Case 4.5. **A,** Expired minute ventilation ($\dot{V}E$) versus oxygen consumption ($\dot{V}O_2$, as a percent of predicted maximum), with predicted line (*dash*) and ventilatory ceiling calculated from $FEV_1 \times 40$. **B,** Workload versus oxygen consumption ($\dot{V}O_2$) with predicted line (*dash*). **C,** Respiratory rate (f) versus tidal volume (VT) with a vertical dashed line representing the patient's vital capacity. **D,** Dead space to tidal volume ratio (VD/VT) versus oxygen consumption ($\dot{V}O_2$, as percent of predicted maximum), with predicted response line (*dash*).

the $PaCO_2$ fell slightly. The AT approximation can be identified by the inflection of the $\dot{V}CO_2$ and $\dot{V}O_2$ graph (Fig. 4.18*D*), but in this patient no inflection upward is seen; therefore, either the AT was not reached or this method of determination was not sensitive enough. Most likely, the AT was not reached.

No abnormalities in the EKG were seen, and the overall impression is that exercise tolerance was severely reduced. Although marked abnormalities of

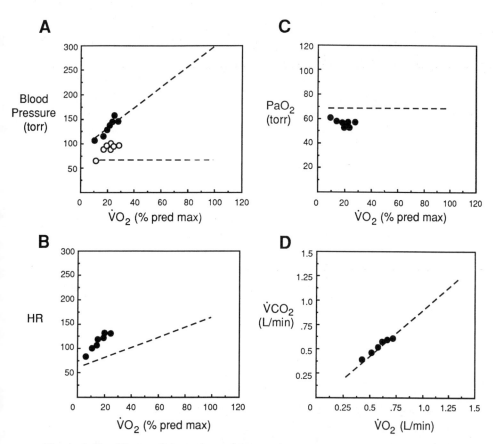

Figure 4.18. The cardiovascular and gas exchange response of the 64-year-old man in Case 4.5. **A,** Systolic (●) and diastolic (O) blood pressure versus oxygen consumption ($\dot{V}O_2$, as a percent of predicted maximum) with normal response lines (*dash*). **B,** Heart rate (HR) versus oxygen consumption ($\dot{V}O_2$, as percent of predicted maximum) with normal response line (*dash*). **C,** PaO_2 versus oxygen consumption ($\dot{V}O_2$, as a percent of predicted maximum) with normal response line (*dash*). **D,** Carbon dioxide production ($\dot{V}CO_2$) versus oxygen consumption ($\dot{V}O_2$) with normal response (*dashed line*) and anaerobic threshold point (AT).

ventilation and gas exchange were present, the patient was not "limited" by these abnormalities. Additionally, the fact that the AT was not achieved suggests deconditioning.

EXERCISE TEST FOR DESATURATION WITH OXIMETRY

The exercise test is particularly useful for evaluation of patients with respiratory disease. The measurement of changes in arterial oxygen levels is used to detect disease, assess severity, and follow changes due to therapy. Additionally, the exercise test and the changes in arterial oxygen are used to assess the need for supplemental oxygen.

The most accurate method of determining arterial oxygen tension (PaO_2) and arterial oxygen saturation (SaO_2) is direct measurement of blood samples taken with a single arterial puncture or an indwelling arterial catheter. However, obtaining the blood sample causes some discomfort, creates risks for the patient, provides only intermittent monitoring, and is costly.

Oximetry devices, on the other hand, are noninvasive, monitor continuously, compare favorably with direct arterial measurements, and are less costly. The devices, which have undergone recent technologic advancements, are becoming increasingly popular. However, their results can sometimes be spurious because of the effects of such factors as skin pigmentation, high carboxy- and methemoglobin levels, nail polish, motion, and ambient light.

This section will discuss the use of pulse oximeters in testing patients with respiratory disease for the evaluation of oxygen desaturation. Because the physiologic response to exercise has previously been discussed, I will focus on patient preparation and testing techniques.

Oximetry

Oximetry is the determination of the percent of hemoglobin that is combined with oxygen. Oximeters use a spectrophotometric technique that measures light absorbance differences between nonoxygenated and oxygenated hemoglobin and apply the principle of the Beer-Lambert-Bouguer law, or simply Beer's law.

Although oximeters were described as early as 1935, it wasn't until the 1960s that Robert Shaw developed the eight-wavelength ear oximeter that was produced by Hewlett-Packard. This device was the first oximeter used extensively in clinical practice. Besides its large size, high cost, and sensitivity to motion artifact, the Hewlett-Packard oximeter could not differentiate between venous and arterial blood. To overcome that problem, the probe (which was designed to fit on the ear) was heated to arterialize the vascular bed of the ear lobe. Additionally, the probe was large, heavy, and uncomfortable to wear.

The **pulse oximeter**, developed in the mid-1970s, measures the change in light transmission in a pulsating area to calculate arterial saturation. For example, if a light source and a detector are placed on opposite sides of a pulsating area (e.g., a finger), a constant amount of light is absorbed by the skin, bone, tissue, and blood. However, when a heartbeat occurs, a small amount of arterial blood increases the blood volume in this area, which re-sults in a change in the light absorption. Therefore, by comparing the pulsa-tile change in light absorption, the absorption of light by skin, bone tissue, and venous blood can be eliminated, isolating arterial blood.

Blood usually contains only two major light absorbers: oxygenated he-moglobin (HbO_2) and nonoxygenated or reduced hemoglobin (RHb). Therefore, only two wavelengths of light are required. By comparing the light absorption of these two wavelengths of light during a heartbeat and between a heartbeat, the ratio of HbO_2 to RHb can be used to determine arterial oxygen saturation.

The lightweight and comfortable probes or cuvettes used with pulse oximeters contain light-emitting diodes (LEDs) and a photodetector. LEDs are available in many wavelengths, but the two most commonly used wave-lengths are 660 and 940 nm. These particular wavelengths distinguish be-tween HbO_2 and RHb extremely well.

The pulse oximeter has been shown to be reasonably accurate,[34-38] but despite its ease of use, portability, and widespread acceptance, the pulse oximeter has some important limitations.

In patients with profound hypoxia (saturations less than 70%), oxime-try has been found to be less reliable.[39,40] In patients undergoing exercise, the pulse oximeter follows the changes in oxygenation reasonably well, but the accuracy has been questioned.[36,41,42]

In addition to problems with severe hypoxia and exercise, pulse ox-imetry is also affected by fingernail polish (when using finger probes), am-bient or fiberoptic light, skin pigmentation, dyes and pigments (e.g., methy-lene blue and bilirubin), and increased levels of other hemoglobins (e.g., carboxyhemoglobin and methemoglobin). The inability to impose quality control against external controls is also an important issue.

The two-sided sensors found in pulse oximetry limit the monitoring sites to either fingers, ears, or toes. However, a single-sided sensor now found in some oximeters uses the methods of light reflectance and back-scattering to transmit and receive the light through any vascular bed. This reflectance oximeter has been found to compare well with other oximeters with regard to time-response and accuracy. However, it may be susceptible to motion artifact.[43]

Patient Preparation

The purpose of this exercise test is to measure changes in arterial oxygen saturation. The patient should take all prescribed medications. The tech-nique described in this section uses a treadmill for the exercise, and the patient should dress appropriately for walking and wear a shirt that allows for easy EKG-lead application.

Testing Technique

The treadmill is recommended (versus free-walking) because it allows for easy EKG, blood pressure, and oximetry monitoring. Additionally, it allows for documentation of workload and better clinical observation by the attending physician and technician. The cycle ergometer is a reasonable alternative, but the treadmill best simulates daily patient activity.

Prior to exercise, the EKG leads should be applied. Twelve leads probably provide better monitoring of EKG changes, but the use of fewer leads is also widely accepted. The resting EKG should be examined for any abnormalities that would contraindicate an exercise test, and a resting blood pressure measurement should be made. The indications to terminate an exercise test listed below also provide contraindications for starting an exercise test.

The pulse oximeter should be applied as described in the instrument's operation manual. There are several different probes (also called cuvettes), and proper placement is critical for accurate readings.

Because the pulse oximeter can be inaccurate, a resting arterial blood gas sample drawn with the oximeter probe properly attached to the patient is recommended. The saturation of the arterial blood gas sample should be determined by CO-oximetry and compared to the pulse oximeter reading (SpO_2) to ensure accuracy.

The patient should have a resting SpO_2 or HbO_2 of 90% or greater. Supplemental O_2 may be necessary to achieve this level. When comparing the arterial blood HbO_2 and the oximeter SpO_2, commonly the SpO_2 is 1 to 4% higher. If the SpO_2 is over 90% and the HbO_2 is less than 90%, the supplemental oxygen flow rate should be adjusted to ensure that the HbO_2 is at least 90%. So, for example, if the HbO_2 is 88% and the SpO_2 is 91% on room air, the O_2 flow rate should be adjusted so that the SpO_2 reads at least 93%. Another blood gas can be obtained to ensure accuracy and ensure that the carbon dioxide tension ($PaCO_2$) has not changed.

Commonly, all of these resting measurements are performed with the patient sitting. However, when the patient stands up, there may be changes in one or several parameters. Therefore, the laboratory should make SpO_2 measurements at rest in both the sitting and standing positions. Allow 1 to 2 minutes of equilibration time with position changes.

Table 4.10: Spirometry results obtained on the 64-year-old man in Case 4.6

	Observed	Predicted	%Predicted
FVC (L)	3.10	5.53	56
FEV$_1$ (L)	1.41	3.77	37
FEV$_1$/FVC (%)	45	68	

The patient should receive instructions from the technician on how to walk on the treadmill prior to the exercise. The treadmill speed should be slow to start, with little or no grade (incline). Many patients with advanced obstructive lung disease are extremely unfit and short of breath, and, thus, speeds of less than 1.5 miles per hour are common. The speed and grade should be increased in small increments up to a level that mimics the exercise levels used by the patient.

The length of time of the exercise period is variable. My recommendation for a maximum time is 6 minutes. If no meaningful desaturation has occurred by that time, the test can be terminated. The test should be terminated in less than 6 minutes if the saturation falls by 5% or falls below 85%.

If the oxygen flow rate required to keep the patient's saturation above a certain level (e.g., 90%) needs to be determined, then one of two approaches can be taken. The first is to exercise the patient and after a meaningful fall in SpO$_2$ (e.g., >5% or below 85%) has occurred, adjust the O$_2$ flow rate while still exercising. However, oftentimes it is difficult to make up the deficit and accurately determine the oxygen flow rate to achieve an appropriate SpO$_2$ level. Therefore, I prefer the second approach, which requires that the technician stop the exercise when a meaningful fall in SpO$_2$ has occurred and adjust the oxygen flow rate to a higher level. After 1 to 3 minutes, when the SpO$_2$ reading has stabilized, restart the exercise and evaluate the new flow rate. If desaturation again occurs, repeat the process of adjusting and reexercising until the 6-minute exercise period or other reasonable time period can be completed without meaningful desaturation or the oxygen flow rates cannot be increased further. I usually do not perform more than three exercise trials at increasing oxygen flow rates without first consulting the ordering physician. This approach can be quite time consuming, but in my opinion it is worth the extra effort.

CASE 4.6

A 64-year-old man was seen in the hospital clinic. He was a new patient and complained of having problems breathing, especially on exertion. Spirometry is

Table 4.11: Arterial blood gas and simultaneous pulse oximeter data on the 64-year-old man in Case 4.6

pH	= 7.42
$PaCO_2$	= 40 mm Hg
PaO_2	= 65 mm Hg*
HbO_2	= 87%†
SpO_2	= 90%

*At sea level
†Measured on CO-oximeter

customarily measured with the first visit; the results are shown in Table 4.10. He claimed to have been a heavy smoker up until 5 years ago when he stopped. He used metaproterenol four times per day and was not on supplementary oxygen. Because he was from out of town and would be staying at a nearby hotel, the physician wanted to determine if he needed supplemental oxygen. Thus, he ordered an exercise test with oximetry and the titration of oxygen to keep the patient's oxygen saturation at 90%.

The patient was escorted to the pulmonary function laboratory, and a 12-lead EKG was applied and a resting blood pressure measured. The EKG was within normal limits and his blood pressure was 138/87 mm Hg. A pulse oximeter was applied using a finger probe and an arterial blood gas sample obtained. The results are shown in Table 4.11.

Question:
How would you proceed?

Answer and Discussion:
Because the arterial saturation measured via the blood sample (HbO_2) was already below 90%, the patient should be placed on oxygen before exercise. One liter/min of oxygen delivered by nasal cannula was applied, and after 5 minutes the SpO_2 was reading 93% (which should produce an HbO_2 of approximately 90%). He got on the treadmill and exercise was started. The SpO_2, which was fluctuating between 89 and 91% at the start, fell to 83 to 85% after 2 minutes of exercise. The treadmill was stopped and the patient was seated.

Question:
What would you do at this point?

Answer and Discussion:
Because the patient is not maintaining an SpO_2 of at least 93%, a higher oxygen flow rate is required and was increased to 2 liters/min. After approximately 5 to

10 minutes, the SpO_2 reading was 94 to 95%, and another exercise period was started. The SpO_2 readings decreased to 91 to 93% over a 6-minute period, and the treadmill was stopped.

Question:
What would you do at this point?

Answer and Discussion:
Because the SpO_2 reading was 3% lower than the blood HbO_2, the goal should be to keep the patients SpO_2 at 93%. This was partially accomplished, but because of the fluctuations in the oximeter readings we cannot be completely sure. It might be appropriate to draw another blood gas to verify the findings. However, practically speaking, the patient remained reasonably oxygenated during exercise when breathing 2 liters/min of nasal oxygen, and therefore no further testing is needed. The physician can be consulted on such questions, but in my experience most physicians would be satisfied at this point.

The physician in this case prescribed home oxygen for this patient—1 liter/min at rest and 2 liters/min when walking.

REFERENCES

1. Jones NL. Clinical exercise testing. 3rd ed. Philadelphia: WB Saunders, 1988.
2. Trautlein JJ. Risk factors in exercise testing. J Allergy Clin Immunol 1979; 64 (part 2):625–626.
3. Jones RS, Buston MH, Wharton MJ. The effect of exercise on ventilatory function in the child with asthma. Br J Dis Chest 1962;56:78–86.
4. Silverman M, Anderson S. Standardization of exercise tests in asthmatic children. Arch Dis Child 1972;47:882–889.
5. Godfrey S. Exercise-induced asthma: clinical, physiological, and therapeutic implications. J Allergy Clin Immunol 1975;56:1–17.
6. Strauss RH, McFadden ER, Ingram RH, Jaeger JJ. Enhancement of exercise-induced asthma by cold air. N Eng J Med 1977;297:743–747.
7. Strauss RH, McFadden ER, Ingram RH, Deal EC, Jaeger JJ. Influence of heat and humidity on the airway obstruction induced by exercise in asthma. J Clin Inv 1978;61:433–440.
8. Bar-Or O, Neuman I, Datan R. Effects of dry and humid climates on exercise-induced asthma in children and pre-adolescents. J Allergy Clin Immunol 1977;60:163–168.
9. McFadden ER, Ingram RH. Exercise-induced asthma; observations on the initiating stimulus. N Eng J Med 1979;301:763–769.
10. Anderson SD, Silverman M, Konig P, Godfrey S. Exercise-induced asthma. Br J Dis Chest 1975;69:1–39.
11. Bierman CW, Spiro SG, Petheram I. Characterization of the late response in exercise-induced asthma. J Allergy Clin Immunol 1984;74:701–706.
12. Zawadski DK, Lenner KA, McFadden ER. Re-examination of the late asthmatic response to exercise. Am Rev Respir Dis 1988;137:837–841.
13. Rubenstein I, Levison H, Slutsky AS, et al. Immediate and delayed bronchoconstriction after exercise in patients with asthma. N Eng J Med 1987;317:482–485.
14. McNeill RS, Nairn JR, Millar JS, Ingram CG. Exercise-induced asthma. Q J Med 1966;35:55–67.

15. Godfrey S, Bar-Yishay E, Ben-Dov I, Springer C. Exercise-induced asthma and the refractory period. Prog Resp Res 1985;19:298–301.

16. Anderson SD, Silverman M, Walker SR. Metabolic and ventilatory changes in asthmatic patients during and after exercise. Thorax 1972;27:718–725.

17. Anderson SA, Seale JP, Ferris L, Schoeffel R, Lindsay DA. An evaluation of pharmacotherapy for exercise-induced asthma. J Allergy Clin Immunology 1979;64:612–624.

18. Anderson SD, Seale JP, Ferris L, Schoeffel R, Lindsay PA. An evaluation of pharmacotherapy for exercise-induced asthma. J Allergy Clin Immunol 1979;64: 612–624.

19. Mellis CM, Kattan M, Keens TG, Levison H. Comparative study of histamine and exercise challenge in asthmatic children. Am Rev Respir Dis 1978;117:911–915.

20. Anderson SD. Exercise-induced asthma: current views. Patient Management 1982; 43–55.

21. Deal EC, McFadden ER, Ingram RH, et al. Airway responsiveness to cold air and hyperpnea in normal subjects and in those with hay fever and asthma. Am Rev Respir Dis 1980;121:621–628.

22. Miller WF, Scacci R, Gast LR. Laboratory evaluation of pulmonary function. Philadelphia: JB Lippincott, 1987:300.

23. Younes M. Interpretation of clinical exercise testing in respiratory disease. Clin Chest Med 1984;5:189–206.

24. Davis FM, Stewart JM. Radial artery cannulation. BR J Anaesth 1980;52:41–47.

25. Gardner RM, Schwartz R, Wong HC, Burke JP. Percutaneous indwelling radial-artery catheters for monitoring cardiovascular function. N Eng J Med 1974; 290:1227–1231.

26. Bedford RF. Radial artery function following percutaneous cannulation with 18 and 20 gauge catheters. Anesthesiology 1977;47:37–39.

27. Jones RM, Hill AB, Nahrwold ML, Bolles RE. The effect of method of radial artery cannulation on post-cannulation blood flow and thrombus formation. Anesthesiology 1981;55:76–78.

28. Bruce RA, McDonough JR. Stress testing in screening for cardiovascular disease. Bull NY Acad Med 1969;45:1288–1305.

29. Nagle FJ, Balke B, Naughton JP. Gradational step tests for assessing work capacity. J Appl Physiol 1965;20:745–748.

30. Sheffield LT, Roitman D. Stress testing methodology. In: Sonnenblick EH, Lasch M, eds., Exercise and heart disease. New York: Green & Stratton, 1977: 145–161.

31. Froelicher VF, Brammel H, Davis G, et al. A comparison of the reproducibility and physiologic response to three maximal treadmill exercise protocols. Chest 1974;65:512–517.

32. Patterson JA, Naughton J, Pietras RJ, Gunnar RM. Treadmill exercise in assessment of the functional capacity of patients with cardiac disease. Am J Cardiol 1972;30:757–762.

33. Jones NL, Makrides L, Hitchcock C, et al. Normal standards for an incremental progressive cycle ergometer test. Am Rev Respir Dis 1985;131:700–708.

34. Rebuk AS, Chapman KR, D'Urzo A. The accuracy and response characteristics of a simplified ear oximeter. Chest 1983; 83:860–864.

35. Shippy MB, Petterson MT, Whitman RA, Shivers CR. A clinical evaluation of the BTI Biox II ear oximeter. Respir Care 1984;29:730–735.

36. Ries AL, Farrow JT, Clausen JL. Accuracy of two ear oximeters at rest and during exercise in pulmonary patients. Am Rev Respir Dis 1985;132:685–689.

37. Cecil WT, Morrison LS, Lamoonpun S. Clinical evaluation of the Ohmeda Biox III pulse oximeter: a comparison of finger and ear cuvettes. Respir Care 1985; 30:840–845.

38. Cecil WT, Thorpe KJ, Fibuch EE, Tuohy GF. A clinical evaluation of the accuracy of the Nellcor N-100 and Ohmeda 3700 pulse oximeters. J Clin Monitoring 1988;4:31–36.

39. Chapman KR, Liu FLW, Watson RM, et al. Range of accuracy of two wave-length oximetry. Chest 1986;89:540–542.

40. Severinghaus JW, Naifeh KH. Accuracy of response of six pulse oximeters to profound hypoxia. Anesthesiology 1987; 67:551–559.
41. Smyth RJ, D'Urzo AD, Slutsky AS, et al. Ear oximetry during combined hypoxia and exercise. J Appl Physiol 1986;60: 716–719.
42. Hansen JE, Casaburi R. Validity of ear oximetry in clinical exercise testing. Chest 1987;91;333–337.
43. Decker MJ, Dickensheets D, Arnold JL, et al. A comparison of a new reflectance oximeter with the Hewlett-Packard ear oximeter. Biomed Instr Tech 1990;24: 122–126.

SELF-ASSESSMENT QUESTIONS

1. All of the following can affect the accuracy of the pulse oximeter except:
   a. profound hypoxemia
   b. exercise
   c. ambient light
   d. bronchodilators
   e. increased carboxyhemoglobin

2. During the first minute of exercise, ventilatory function as measured by PEFR usually:
   a. increases
   b. decreases
   c. cannot be measured
   d. none of above

3. A standardized time for an exercise period when evaluating a patient for exercise-induced asthma is:
   a. 1 to 2 minutes
   b. 6 to 8 minutes
   c. 13 to 15 minutes
   d. 20 to 22 minutes

4. Which of the following forms of exercise are considered to be the most asthmogenic?
   a. running
   b. swimming
   c. walking
   d. cycling

5. All of the following are considered to be factors in producing exercise-induced asthma except:
   a. age
   b. heat and moisture loss

c. intensity of exercise

d. mechanical stimulation of breathing at high minute ventilation

6. During a maximum workload symptom-limited exercise test, minute ventilation in a normal individual:

a. increases in a nonlinear fashion

b. increases in a linear fashion up to approximately 50% of maximum VO_2

c. increases up to the ventilatory ceiling

d. both a and c

e. both b and c

7. The main cardiovascular response to exercise is:

a. increase in ventilation

b. increase in cardiac output

c. increase in blood pressure

d. decrease in arterial oxygen content

8. All of the following are characteristics of the breath-by-breath method of exercise measurements except:

a. rapid response gas analyzers

b. computerization

c. 3-liter mixing chamber

d. synchronization of gas analyzer and volume signals

9. During exercise, the oxygen consumption increases with work:

a. in a linear fashion

b. in a nonlinear fashion

c. does not increase with work

d. only when PaO_2 increases

10. The respiratory quotient (R) measures the relationship of:

a. CO_2 production to CO_2 consumption

b. CO_2 production to O_2 production

c. CO_2 production to O_2 consumption

d. CO_2 production to minute ventilation

11. A patient's resting blood pressure is 120/65. After 4 minutes of exercise, the blood pressure is 190/70. This is:

a. a normal response

b. a hypotensive response

    c. a hypertensive response

    d. an indication to stop the exercise test

12. In healthy individuals the dead space to tidal volume (V_D/V_T) ratio is:

    a. 0.35 at rest and decreases with exercise

    b. 0.35 at rest and increases with exercise

    c. 0.50 at rest and is unchanged with exercise

    d. 0.50 at rest and decreases with exercise

5

Methacholine and Histamine Bronchial Provocation Tests

The evaluation of "twitchy" or hyperresponsive airways is an increasingly popular but difficult task for the pulmonary function laboratory. The test is frequently called a "challenge" and uses a stimulant to provoke airway changes. A number of stimuli can be used including exercise, cold air, occupational exposures, and a group of aerosolized substances (e.g., methacholine, histamine, carbochol, antigen, and distilled water). A number of techniques exist for using each stimulant, but unfortunately, no agreement has been reached on which stimulant or technique best evaluates hyperresponsiveness. Additionally, technicians may be apprehensive because the tests can cause adverse reactions and because they are done infrequently.

This chapter focuses on the use of aerosolized methacholine and histamine because they are the most commonly used substances, have somewhat standardized procedures, and are easy to perform. Additionally, they are believed to be useful and safe.

INDICATIONS

Reasons for Performing Bronchial Challenges

One reason for performing bronchial challenges is to **diagnose asthma**. Because asthma is characterized by hyperresponsive airways, distinguishing between hyperresponsive and normal airways is important. Many patients with normal pulmonary function test results and little or no response to bronchodilators have complaints of "tightness," wheezing, or isolated coughing.

Members of another group of patients demonstrate spirometric improvement after use of a bronchodilator or have diurnal variation in peak flows. In this group, the indication for bronchial challenges is to **confirm a diagnosis of asthma**.

Another indication for bronchial challenge is to **document the severity** of hyperresponsiveness by determining the precise concentration that causes a clinically important fall in pulmonary function. A large difference in the perception of "tightness" or wheezing exists among patients and/or their parents—a difference that can interfere with subjective evaluation and increase the need for objective data.

Following changes in hyperresponsiveness is yet another indication for a bronchial challenge. Changes in medication regimens can increase or decrease the level of hyperresponsiveness. Additionally, increases or decreases in occupational exposure can also lead to changes in hyperresponsiveness. Finally, in looking toward the future, I anticipate the use of bronchial challenges in the workplace as a screening test to identify workers who may be at risk.

Summary of indications for methacholine/histamine challenges

---

1. *Diagnose asthma*
2. *Confirm a diagnosis of asthma*
3. *Document the severity of hyperresponsiveness*
4. *Follow changes in hyperresponsiveness*

PHYSIOLOGY

When certain pharmacologic agents (e.g., methacholine and histamine) are inhaled by patients with hyperresponsive airways, the airways respond by constricting or narrowing. In order to understand this action, let us first look at the physiology of airway smooth muscle innervation.

The human nervous system is divided into two parts: (*a*) the central nervous system, which consists of the brain and spinal cord, and (*b*) the peripheral nervous system, which contains nerves including the vagus that connect the central system to all other parts of the body.

The peripheral nervous system includes the autonomic nerves—branches of certain cranial and spinal nerves that innervate organs in the thorax, abdomen, pelvis, and most of the blood vessels and glands in the body.

The autonomic system is essentially a two-cell and two-fiber system. The originating neuron cell starts in the gray matter of the brain or spinal cord, and then a preganglionic fiber extends to a ganglion. From the ganglion, a second neuron cell makes its synapse with the preganglionic fiber, and a postganglionic fiber extends to the part it innervates (neuroeffector junction). This system is illustrated in Figure 5.1.

The transmission of signals through the synapses of the autonomic system is mediated by two chemicals (or neurotransmitters): acetylcholine and norepinephrine.

The autonomic system is divided into the sympathetic and parasympathetic divisions. The sympathetic division (also called the adrenergic system) involves both acetylcholine and norepinephrine. At the ganglion, acetylcholine is the mediator, but at the neuroeffector junction, norepinephrine is the mediator.

The parasympathetic (also called cholinergic) division of the autonomic system is concerned with processes that conserve energy and generally inhibit or slow activities of organs. The transmission of signals from the vagus nerves through the synapse at both the ganglion (located in the walls of the airway) and neuroeffector junctions is mediated by the production of acetylcholine (cholinergic action)

The epithelium of the conducting airways consists of ciliated pseudo-stratified columnar epithelial cells, mucosal glands, receptor cells, and bronchial smooth muscle. Figure 5.2 is a simplified drawing showing the epithelial cells lining the airway lumen and the receptor cells (irritant cells). Signals from these receptor cells travel to the brain via the vagus afferent pathway.

Histamine produces two actions. The first is the stimulation of the irritant cells. The resulting signal travels to the brain (via the afferent pathway). From the brain, the return signal travels down the vagus to the preganglionic fibers (efferent pathway) leading to the ganglion through acetylcholine mediation. From the ganglion, the signal travels to the neuroeffector junction (airway smooth muscle), where again acetylcholine is released and combines with muscarinic receptors in the smooth muscle and contraction takes place (Fig. 5.2). This reflexive action is blocked by atropine (an anticholinergic).[1]

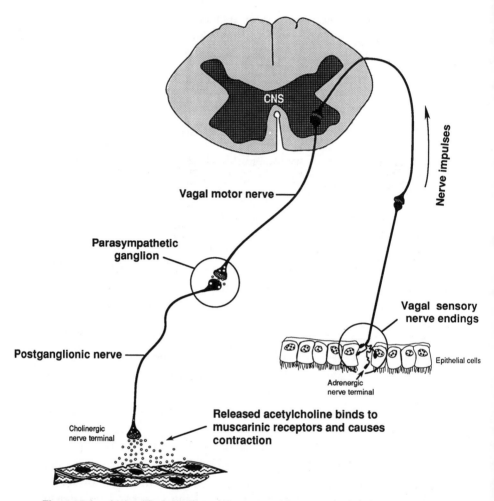

Figure 5.1. A simplified drawing of the autonomic nervous system as it applies to innervation of bronchial smooth muscle. Impulses from receptor cells in the airway are sent to the central nervous system (CNS). From the CNS the impulse travels to the parasympathetic ganglion, to the postganglionic neuron, and ultimately to the nerve terminal (neuroeffector junction) where acetylcholine is released and combines with muscle receptors.

The second action of histamine is directly on the smooth muscle. Histamine diffuses through airway cells to the muscle where it combines with H_1 receptors, causing contraction.

Methacholine's action is similar to the second action of histamine in that it diffuses to the muscle and causes direct contraction without nervous

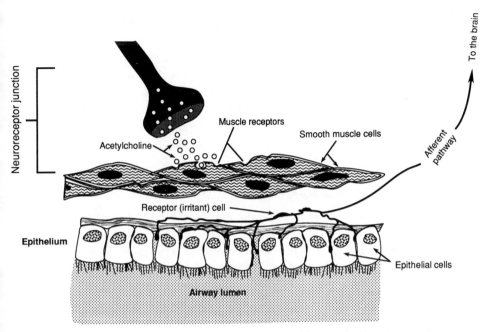

Figure 5.2. A simplified drawing of the epithelium of the conducting airways showing the receptor cells and subsequent innervation of the smooth muscle via cholinergic action.

activity. This raises the possibility that some airways could be responsive to histamine and not to methacholine.

METHACHOLINE VS. HISTAMINE VS. EXERCISE

Exercise-induced asthma (discussed in Chapter 4) is found in 70 to 80% of asthmatics[2] and therefore has been used as a method to make or confirm the diagnosis of asthma. However, when compared to the methods using methacholine or histamine, exercise, despite being more natural, has not been found to be a particularly good test.[3-8] I have seen a few cases where challenge to methacholine was negative, but to exercise it was positive. These cases were puzzling, and I wanted to retest the patients to verify the results. But, for various reasons I was not able to do so. Therefore, questions such as whether or not patient preparation was appropriate (e.g., medications not held) or whether there were problems with the reagents or the nebulizer were not answered.

The results of challenges with methacholine and histamine have good correlation and reproducibility.[9] It is generally agreed that similar concentrations of histamine and methacholine produce similar results in asthmatics. For example, equal doses (e.g., 2.5 mg/ml) of methacholine and histamine produce similar changes in pulmonary function test results in a given patient. Methacholine, however, has been shown to better differentiate asthmatics from normal subjects.[4,10] Histamine is associated with more side effects (e.g., throat irritation, flushing, and headaches) especially at higher doses, and some asthmatics have developed a tolerance and have become unresponsive to the higher doses.[11,12] Consequently, methacholine has become the agent of preference in clinical practice.

OBTAINING AND STORING THE AGENTS

Methacholine chloride seems to be the more difficult to obtain. However, one product (Provocholine, Roche Laboratories) is now readily available in easy-to-dilute vials. If methacholine is obtained in bulk dry powder, it must be stored in a dessicant container and kept in the freezer. After it has been diluted, it has been shown to be stable for at least 4 months when stored at approximately 4°C.[13,14] For Provocholine, the company recommends only a 2-week storage time of the higher concentrations and immediate discard of the lowest concentration after use.

Histamine acid phosphate can also be obtained in a powder form. After dilution, it is stable for many months.

Methacholine and histamine are mixed in a solution called the "diluent." The recommended diluent consists of 0.5% NaCl, 0.275% $NaHCO_3$, and 0.4% phenol[15] and can be obtained from Hollister Stier (Miles Inc., Pharmaceuticals Division; Spokane, WA).

DOSING AND DELIVERY TECHNIQUES

Once the challenge material has been obtained and properly stored, a very critical step must be taken—making the dilutions and delivering the solution to the patient.

Dilution of products such as Provocholine is simple and well described in the product insert. However, measuring bulk powders and diluting them is much more difficult and is best done by the hospital pharmacist. Once diluted, the reagent vials or bottles should be labeled, dated, and stored in the refrigerator.

One frequently used dosing schedule[16] is:

Methacholine (mg/ml)	Histamine (mg/ml)
0.075	0.03
0.15	0.06

0.31	0.12
0.62	0.25
1.25	1.0
2.5	2.5
5.0	5.0
10.0	10.0
25.0	

Another dosing schedule[17] that uses the same dosing for both methacholine and histamine is:

0.03 mg/ml
0.06
0.125
0.25
0.50
1.0
2.0
4.0
8.0
16.0

The formulation of these schedules was largely the result of the concentration available from the chemical suppliers.

The reader should note from these dosing schedules that the concentration of the challenge agent is slowly increased in a systematic manner. Such slow increases not only are safer but also allow for better interpretation of results.

Getting the challenge material from the nebulizer to the airway is important and appears simple; as an example one might only have to put 1 or 2 cc of each dose in a nebulizer and have the patient inhale a set number of breaths. But, it is not quite that simple when one considers the many factors affecting the amount of challenge material that reaches the airway.

The amount reaching the mouth from the nebulizer is dependent on such things as:

Nebulizer output;
Particle size;
Amount/type of tubing between nebulizer and mouth;
Continuous versus intermittent aerosol;
Amount of liquid in nebulizer.

Reaching the smooth muscles of the airway from the mouth is dependent not only on the just mentioned factors but also on such factors as:

Inspiratory flow rate;
Lung volume at beginning of inspiration;
Breathing pattern;
Particle size;
Volume inhaled;
Breathhold time.

This chapter will not discuss the issues surrounding all of these factors; however, one of the most important factors, nebulizer output, deserves some discussion. It makes sense that the more output from the nebulizer, the more challenge material potentially available to travel to the airway smooth muscle. Ryan and coworkers[18] have demonstrated a wide range of outputs among various brands at the same flow rate and that the output of a particular nebulizer varies directly with the powering flow rate (Fig. 5.3). A study of the reproducibility of nebulizer output has shown the coefficient of variation to be 24% for numerous nebulizers of the same brand and 10% for repeated measurements of the same nebulizer.[19]

Output measurement simply requires that the nebulizer be accurately weighed before and after nebulizing water or saline for a known period of time. I have found it helpful to nebulize for 4 or 5 minutes to ensure a representative per-minute measurement.

Delivery Techniques

The two most widely used and accepted methods of delivery are (*a*) the 2-minute tidal breathing method and (*b*) the five-deep-breath method.

Cockcroft and coworkers[17] have described a 2-minute tidal breathing technique that uses a low-output nebulizer (Wright). For 2 minutes at resting tidal volume and rate, the patient breathes the aerosol from a face mask held over the mouth and with the nose clipped.

The Wright nebulizer (Fig. 5.4) is expensive ($90) and sometimes difficult to obtain because it is made only in Canada and England. The output of this nebulizer is approximately 0.13 to 0.16 ml/min when powered at a flow rate of 7 to 8 liters/min. By contrast, the DeVilbiss* 645 nebulizer (Fig. 5.5) has an output of approximately 0.25 ml/min when powered by the same flow rate. One could use a DeVilbiss type nebulizer in place of the Wright

---

*DeVilbiss Health Care, Inc., Somerset, PA.

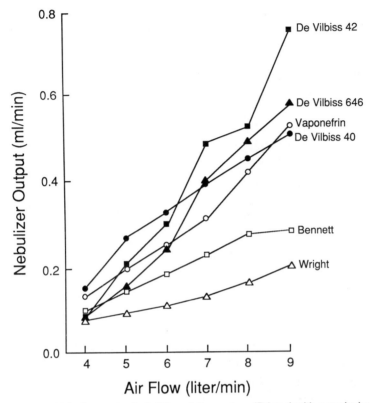

Figure 5.3. Nebulizer output at different flow rates. (Printed with permission from Ryan G, et al. Standardization of inhalation provocation tests: influence of nebulizer output, particle size, and method of inhalation. Ryan G, Dolovich MB, Obminski G, et al. J Allergy Clin Immunol 1981;67:156–161.)

for this technique, but the powering flow rate would have to be lower (e.g., 4 to 5 liters/min) to produce the desired 0.13 to 0.16 ml/min output.

The second delivery technique (five-deep-breath method) was recommended by Chai and coworkers[16] and has the patient take five consecutive deep breaths from functional residual capacity (FRC) to total lung capacity (TLC) using a **dosimeter** (Fig. 5.6). Inspiration should be prolonged (i.e., 1 to 5 sec) with a short breathhold of approximately 2 to 5 seconds.[20] The dosimeter has an electrically controlled valve that can be opened for variable amounts of time. It requires a pressurized gas source and is usually used with a DeVilbiss 646 nebulizer (Fig. 5.5), which has two large openings—one for the patient to inhale from and the second to house a sensing device to activate the dosimeter. Dosimeters are expensive (approximately

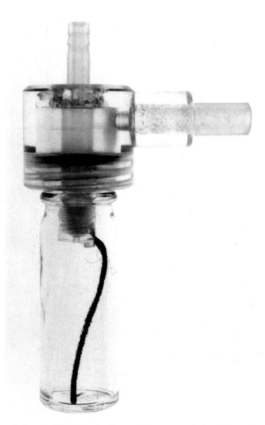

Figure 5.4.   A Wright nebulizer. (Photograph by Barry Silverstein.)

$1200 to $2000). One type (French-Rosenthal) can be ordered from Johns Hopkins University.

The 2-minute method and the dosimeter five-deep-breath method have produced similar results and reproducibility.[20]

A variation of the five-deep-breath technique is to inhale five consecutive deep breaths from FRC to TLC in the same manner as above but without the dosimeter. Most laboratories cannot justify the cost of a dosimeter if challenges are done infrequently. I have used this "no-dosimeter" technique and compared results with results obtained with the dosimeter technique and have found the two to produce similar results (i.e., the concentration causing a significant fall in ventilatory function is similar). Yan and coworkers[21] also compared the results of a "no-dosimeter" technique (hand-operated nebulizer) to those of a dosimeter technique and found no significant difference.

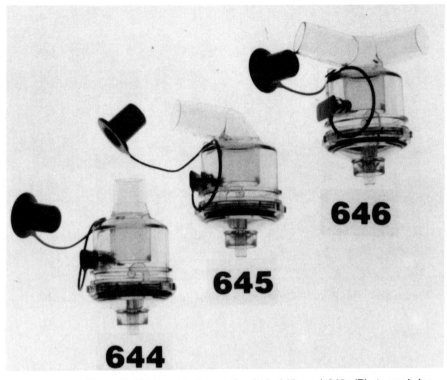

646

645

644

Figure 5.5. Three DeVilbiss nebulizers—the 644, 645, and 646. (Photograph by Barry Silverstein.)

Starting Dose

Regardless of the aerosol generation or delivery method used, the starting dose should be very low (e.g., 0.03 to 0.15 mg/ml) when patients suspected of being hyperresponsive are being tested. After the initial dose, concentrations should be increased one step at a time (usually a twofold increment) until the test is positive or the highest dose is reached.

Methods that employ higher initial doses have been described. The American Thoracic Society (ATS)[15] states that when the purpose is to determine whether a patient has hyperresponsive airways, the challenge may be performed in one to two doses. The initial dose should be one to which normal subjects do not usually respond (i.e., less than 8 mg/ml). Additional doses are given when no response has occurred to the first.

Chatham and coworkers[22] described a shortened test using the ATS recommendations—one breath of 5 mg/ml followed by four additional

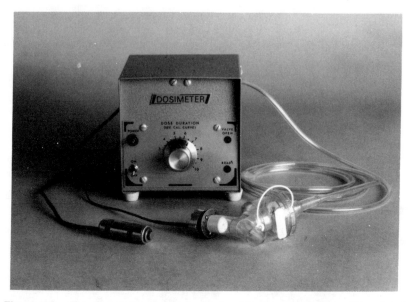

Figure 5.6. The French-Rosenthal dosimeter. (Photograph by Barry Silverstein.)

breaths of 5 mg/ml of methacholine, then one breath of 25 mg/ml, and finally four breaths of 25 mg/ml. There were 5-minute intervals between inhalations, during which spirometry was measured.

Corrao[23] describes another "quickie" approach: one breath of 25 mg/ml. If after 5 minutes the FEV_1 does not fall by more than 20%, then give four additional breaths of the same concentration.

Finally, Hargreave[9] has offered some helpful guidelines to help shorten the study time. If the patient's FEV_1 is more than 80% of predicted and does not fall by more than 10% after diluent, and if the patient is on no pulmonary medications, the starting dose can be as high as 1 to 2 mg/ml. If the patient is on bronchodilators, the starting dose should be 0.25 mg/ml, and if the patient is on steroids, the starting dose should be 0.125 mg/ml. In all other instances, the starting concentration should be 0.03 mg/ml.

The laboratory should be consistent in delivery method and dosing schedule, and I recommend that the delivery technique be noted in the report. As a quality-control mechanism, nebulizer outputs should be checked periodically, and, because of internebulizer variability, the same nebulizer should be used for repeat studies of the same patient.

PATIENT PREPARATION

Bronchial challenges require special attention to patient preparation. If the patient has not been prepared properly or is doing poorly, the challenge should be postponed. The more important patient preparation factors include medications, viral infections, smoking, antigen exposures, and suggestion. In addition, contraindication criteria should be established to determine if a challenge can be carried out.

Factors in Patient Preparation

1. **Medications.** Withhold all medications if possible. If all medications cannot be withheld for the recommended period of time, the challenge can still be done but with the knowledge of what medications the patient took. Check with the ordering doctor to determine if it is acceptable to proceed. In 1980, the ATS suggested the following schedule for withholding medications prior to challenges[15]:

   Inhaled bronchodilators: 4 to 12 hours, depending on specific drug's duration of action.

   Oral bronchodilators: 12 to 18 hours for short-acting theophylline preparations
   24 to 28 hours for long-acting theophylline preparations

   Antihistamines: 48 hours

   Cromolyn Sodium: 48 hours

   Hydroxyzine: 96 hours

   The European Society of Clinical Respiratory Physiology (SECPR) also suggested some guidelines on withholding medications in 1983[24]

   β2-adrenergic agonist aerosols: 12 hours

   Anticholinergic aerosols: 12 hours

   Cromolyn Sodium: 8 hours

   β2-adrenergic agonists (oral): 12 hours

   Theophyllines: 48 hours

   H_1-receptor antagonists: 48 hours

   Because of the large amount of research activity in bronchial reactivity and its mechanisms, updates on these guidelines are probably needed.

2. **Cola drinks, chocolate, and smoking.** The ATS recommends that these be voided for at least 2 hours prior to the challenge.

3. **Viral infections.** Infections can increase hyperresponsiveness of the airways for as long as 3 weeks and therefore are a valid reason to be considered as a criterion for postponing the challenge.

4. **Antigen and occupational exposures.** These can also increase airway hyperresponsiveness and should be avoided for at least 24 hours.

5. **Suggestion.** Both bronchoconstriction and bronchodilatation can be induced by suggestion.[25,26] One study found that bronchodilatation or constriction can be accomplished in 47.5% of asthmatic subjects with appropriate suggestion.[27] Therefore, it is best to tell the patient as little as possible. However, most patients want to know what is involved and can be told that they will be inhaling some aerosols (mists) that can make them worse or better or cause no change. **Avoid giving them too much information.**

When the patient comes to the laboratory, baseline pulmonary function tests should be done. The laboratory should have some contraindication criteria in place to alert the technician that the patient may not be fit to challenge today. In my opinion, adults with FEV_1s <1.5 liters and children with FEV_1s <1.0 liter are not good candidates for a challenge for two major reasons: (*a*) Small changes in FEV_1 yield large percent changes (i.e., just the variability between efforts can lead to a questionable interpretation), and (*b*) there is little room to fall. In these situations, the physician should be consulted to determine if the challenge should be performed.

In addition, an FEV_1 of less than 70% of a patient's best prebronchodilator value within the last 3 months should also raise concern. It indicates that the patient may be doing poorly today, and the ordering physician should be consulted as to whether the challenge should be performed.

One other contraindication criterion should be considered. On occasion, the FEV_1 will change (increase or decrease) after inhalation of the diluent alone. If the FEV_1 *increases* by more than 10%, it is recommended that the technician administer another diluent and remeasure PFTs to ensure a consistent and known starting point. If after the inhalation of the diluent the FEV_1 *falls* 10 to 20%, another diluent should be administered and PFTs remeasured. If the FEV_1 *falls by another 10%*, or more than a total of 20% after diluent, the challenge probably should be postponed because the patient is too responsive at the time.

Laboratory safety is an issue that comes up from time to time. In my opinion, a physician does not need to present. The technicians should be knowledgeable of therapeutic procedures for respiratory dysfunction (i.e., bronchodilator and oxygen therapy) and should have cardiopulmonary resuscitation (CPR) certification. It is my experience that methacholine and histamine challenges are safe and do not require extensive safety requirements.

The room in which the challenge is performed should be well ventilated. In my opinion there is not a need for exhausting excess aerosol to the outside or through exotic filtering systems. Technicians with asthma or other respiratory problems should avoid performing this test.

PULMONARY FUNCTION TESTS

To be useful for diagnosis and management, response to bronchial challenge must be measured as change or lack of change in pulmonary function. Simple spirometry produces FEV_1 and FEF25-75%; the body box and other devices produce airways resistance and specific conductance by panting or quiet breathing. But (*a*) What measurements are best? (*b*) How much change is required to be meaningful? (*c*) When are the measurements made? and (*d*) How is change calculated?

To recognize hyperresponsive airways, spirometry is usually sufficient. The ATS recommends that FEV_1 be included in all bronchial challenge tests, even if other values are measured and reported.[15] However, FEV_1 may not be the most sensitive measurement, and because changes in FVC are usually similar to those for FEV_1, the FEV_1/FVC % ratio is not a useful measurement.

However, in some cases, spirometry may be undesirable in bronchial challenges. For example, the deep breath required to perform spirometry can cause bronchodilatation, and multiple spirometric efforts can cause bronchoconstriction.

By using the panting maneuver in a body box or quiet breathing on some newer devices, one can measure airways resistance and specific conductance without the necessity for a deep breath. However, these instruments are expensive and more complicated to operate. Thus, most laboratories do not invest in them.

According to the ATS,[15] the minimum acceptable changes that define a positive test for three commonly measured values are:

$FEV_1 = -20\%$
FEF25-75% $= -25\%$
SGaw $= -40\%$

Knowing when to make measurements and which effort in a group of efforts to report is critical. Methacholine and histamine are fast acting and usually reach maximal effect in 1 to 5 minutes, plateau, and then quickly lose their effect. The plateau duration is approximately 4 and 12 minutes, which means that the assessment should be made within this time after the end of nebulization.[28] However, there may be increased variability in the pulmonary function measurements because of this time course. For example, after a specific dose, the FEV_1 may be lowest on the first effort and increase with each subsequent effort or vice versa. So which FEV_1 do you report for a given dose? You may choose either (*a*) the lowest and most reproducible FEV_1 values, or (*b*) the highest FEV_1, or (*c*) the FEV_1 from the best effort (highest sum). But **be consistent and note the basis for your choice.**

Once the decision is made on which FEV_1 to use, calculation of the percent change is easy. Use the highest, lowest, or most reproducible post diluent (saline) value and the corresponding postchallenge material value as shown in the following example:

DOSE (mg/ml)	FEV, Effort (L)		
	1	2	3
Baseline	3.20	3.24	3.30
Diluent	3.27	3.24	3.29
0.31 mg/ml	2.94	2.98	3.03

using the lowest FEV_1 values:

$$\% \text{ Change} = \frac{\text{lowest postdiluent} - \text{lowest postmethacholine}}{\text{lowest postdiluent}}$$

$$= \frac{3.24 - 2.94}{3.24} = -9.3\%$$

or, using the highest FEV_1 values:

$$\% \text{ Change} = \frac{\text{highest postdiluent} - \text{highest postmethacholine}}{\text{highest postdiluent}}$$

$$= \frac{3.29 - 3.03}{3.29} = -7.9\%$$

If you are reporting specific conductance (SGaw), a mean of several trials for each dose is usually reported. The calculation of the percent change is then done in the manner above.

EXPRESSING THE RESULTS

There are number of ways to express the results from a methacholine or histamine challenge. For example, the dose can be expressed as cumulative or noncumulative units, as micromoles (which includes nebulizer output), or as dose concentration expressed in mg/ml or breath units. Conse-

	Baseline	Diluent	0.31	0.62	1.25	2.50	Rx
FVC (L)	5.75	5.71	5.69	5.68	5.24	4.93	5.70
FEV$_1$ (L)	4.31	4.29	4.21	4.09	3.79	3.29	4.20
FEV$_1$ /FVC (%)	75	75	74	72	72	67	74
% Change FEV$_1$*	—	—	-2	-5	-12	-23	

* Percent change from diluent

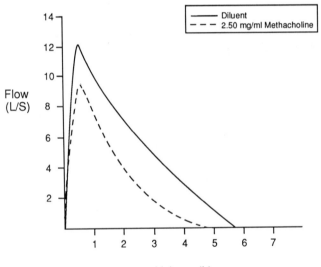

Figure 5.7. Tabular format of a typical methacholine challenge and flow-volume curves of the diluent and the dose that caused a greater than 20% fall in FEV$_1$ (2.5 mg/ml).

quently, the variety of methods creates a problem of making comparisons between studies.

Figures 5.7 and 5.8 report histamine or methacholine test information in tabular and graphic format. Figure 5.7 gives the pulmonary function values for baseline, diluent, and each dose and representative flow-volume curves for diluent and the dose that casued more than a 20% fall in FEV$_1$.

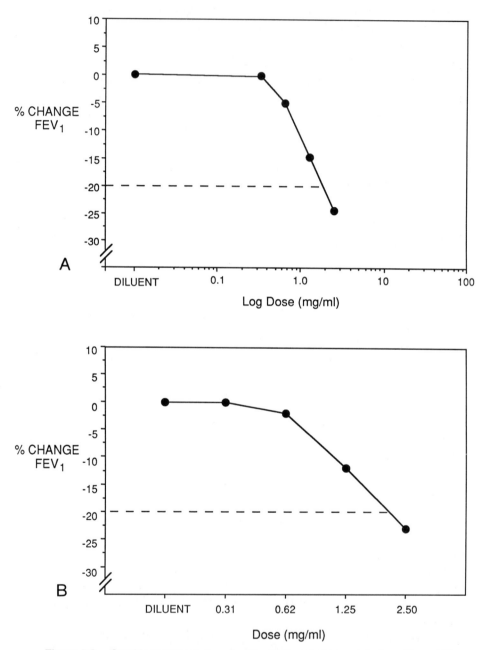

Figure 5.8. Graphic representation of methacholine challenge data from Figure 5.7. Figure 5.8*A* uses the noncumulative log dose in mg/ml for the X-axis, and Figure 5.8*B* uses the dose in mg/ml for its X-axis.

Figure 5.8 displays two ways of graphically displaying the challenge. Figure 5.8A plots percent change in FEV_1 on the Y-axis and noncumulative log dose in mg/ml on the X-axis. Figure 5.8B plots percent change in FEV_1 on the Y-axis and the dose administered in mg/ml on the X-axis.

The position, slope, and shape of the graphic format's curve have been looked at in a number of ways. However, the most common method of analysis is by calculation of the provocative dose (PD), also called "provocative concentration" (PC), the dose that causes a meaningful fall in a pulmonary function parameter and displayed as in Figure 5.9. For example, $PC_{20}FEV_1$ refers to the provocative concentration that caused a 20% fall in FEV_1; $PC_{40}SGaw$ refers to the provocative concentration that caused a 40% fall in specific conductance.

The calculation of the PC or PD is done by linear interpolation. Many pulmonary function testing instruments today have programs that do this automatically. However, the process is relatively simple by hand as demonstrated in the following example.

METHACHOLINE DOSE	FEV₁ Effort (L)			%CHANGE
	1	2	3	
Baseline	4.28	4.31	4.27	
Diluent	4.24	4.21	4.29	
0.31 mg/ml	4.18	4.14	4.21	2*
0.62	4.04	4.09	4.08	5
1.25	3.79	3.74	3.76	12
2.50	3.24	3.27	3.29	23

*The highest FEV_1 at each dose was used, and percent change calculated from postdiluent FEV_1.

Calculations:

Using the linear interpolation formula of:

$$\frac{X - X_1}{Y - Y_1} = \frac{X_2 - X_1}{Y_2 - Y_1}$$

Where $X = PC_{20}FEV_1$; $X_1 =$ log dose preceding the dose that caused a 20% fall; $X_2 =$ log dose that caused a 20% fall; $Y = 80\%$ of postdiluent FEV_1; $Y_1 = FEV_1$ of dose preceding the dose that caused a 20% fall; $Y_2 = FEV_1$ of dose that caused a 20% fall.

Simplifying:

$$\log X = \log X_1 + \frac{(Y - Y_1)(X_2 - X_1)}{(Y_2 - Y_1)}$$

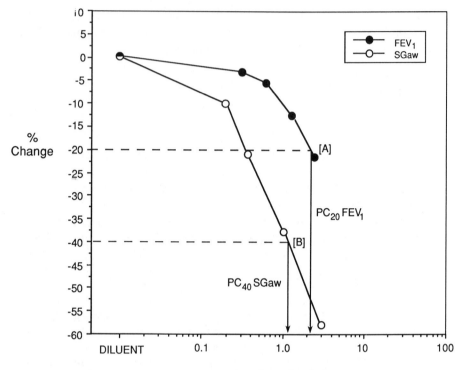

Figure 5.9. Graphic representation of methacholine data from Figure 5.7. The solid circles show FEV_1, and the open circles show specific conductance (SGaw). A 20% fall in FEV_1 is generally considered to be meaningful, and a dashed line extends from -20% on the Y-axis to the FEV_1 line and intersects it at point A, from which a vertical line ($PC_{20}FEV_1$) points to the precise concentration on the X-axis. Similarly, a 40% fall in SGaw is considered to be meaningful, and a dashed line extends from -40% on the Y-axis to the SGaw line and intersects it at point B, from which a vertical line ($PC_{40}SGaw$) points to the precise concentration on the X-axis.

$$\log PC_{20}FEV_1 = \log 1.25 + \frac{(3.43 - 3.79)(\log 2.5 - \log 1.25)}{(3.29 - 3.79)}$$

$$\log PC_{20}FEV_1 = 0.097 + \frac{(-0.36)(0.398 - 0.097)}{-0.50}$$

$$\log PC_{20}FEV_1 = 0.097 + 0.217$$
$$\log PC_{20}FEV_1 = 0.314$$
$$PC_{20}FEV_1 = 2.07 \text{ mg/ml}$$

PROCEDURE

The basic procedure for performing methacholine or histamine bronchial challenges is the same.

1. Ensure proper patient preparation as discussed above.
2. Explain the procedure, but avoid giving too much information.
3. Obtain baseline pulmonary function tests (PFTs) and check for any contra-indications.
4. Aerosolize the diluent (saline) in the same manner that the challenge material will be aerosolized, and have the patient inhale the specified number of breaths or breathe for the specified period of time.
5. Begin the PFTs approximately 1 to 3 minutes (keep this time constant) after diluent administration. It is important that the diluent not cause significant bronchoconstriction or bronchodilatation. Therefore, if FEV_1 *falls* or *increases* by 10 to 20%, another diluent should be administered and PFTs remeasured. If after the second diluent the FEV_1 falls by another 10%, the challenge should be postponed. Likewise, if the FEV_1 falls by more than 20% after the first or subsequent diluent inhalations, the challenge should be postponed.
6. Have the patient inhale the lowest or first concentration of challenge material according to the laboratory's dosing schedule. Wait 1 to 3 minutes and begin the PFTs in the same manner as was done after administration of the diluent. If the FEV_1 falls less than 20%, give the next strongest dose.
7. Continue the challenge until the FEV_1 has fallen by 20% or until the highest concentration has been inhaled.
8. Administer an aerosolized bronchodilator after a positive response has been obtained (i.e., a 20% fall in FEV_1).

BASIC ELEMENTS OF INTERPRETATION

Elements to be included in the interpretation of histamine and methacholine challenges depend in part on the reason for performing the challenge. If the purpose is to confirm a diagnosis of asthma, then the presence of hyperresponsiveness with the specific provocative concentrations should be noted in the interpretation. On the other hand, if the reason for the challenge is to follow changes in hyperresponsiveness, then the interpretation may be more complex and include not only the change in the PC_{20} or in the shape of the dose-response curve from the previous test but also comments on reactivity (slope of the dose-response curve) and sensitivity (the horizontal placement of the PC_{20}).

The reaction of normal populations to methacholine and histamine is somewhat variable. This is due to the fact that uniform standardization of methodology has not been achieved. However, in the most commonly used techniques described earlier, the range of the lower limit of normal re-

Table 5.1: Spirometry before and after bronchodilator on the 10-year-old boy in Case 5.1

	Pre-RX	Post-RX
FVC (L)	2.50 (128)*	2.72
FEV_1 (L)	2.00 (114)	2.31
FEV_1/FVC (%)	80	85

*Values in parentheses are percent predicted.

sponse for $PC_{20}FEV_1$ is 4 to 16 mg/ml (noncumulative) and 40 to 160 cumulative breath units. In unpublished studies of laboratory workers I found that normals did not have $PC_{20}FEV_1$s lower than 16 mg/ml of methacholine; however, I usually use a $PC_{20}FEV_1$ of 8 mg/ml as the dividing point between hyperresponsive and normal airways.

Hargreave[29] used the following guidelines for defining hyperresponsiveness and describing the severity of the reaction.

$PC_{20}FEV_1$ (mg/ml)	Severity
0.03–0.124	Severe
0.125–1.99	Moderate
2.00–7.99	Mild
Above 8.00	Normal

CASE 5.1

A 10-year-old boy with a history of coughing after gym class was sent to the pulmonary function laboratory for a methacholine challenge. Pulmonary function results from an earlier visit are shown in Table 5.1 and Figure 5.10.

The methacholine challenge results are shown in Table 5.2 and Figure 5.11.

Questions:
1. What is the interpretation of the methacholine challenge?
2. What suggestion could be made to testing laboratory?

Answers and Discussion:
The methacholine challenge is positive, as the FEV_1 fell by more than 20% at a moderately low dose. The $PC_{20}FEV_1$ of 1.10 mg/ml suggests a mild to moderate sensitivity.

The issue with this challenge is that the patient's FEV_1 fell more than 20% on the first dose of methacholine administered. Thus, is the first dose too high? Yes, it is, and the laboratory should consider a dosing schedule that begins at less concentrated doses. However, laboratories use a variety of dosing sched-

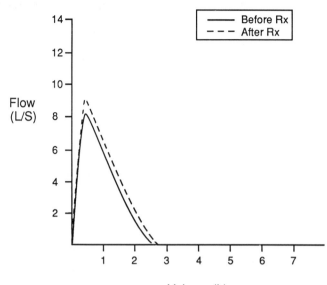

Figure 5.10. Flow-volume curves before and after bronchodilator (RX) on the 10-year-old boy in Case 5.1.

Table 5.2: Results from methacholine challenge showing FEV$_1$ and percent change from diluent

	FEV$_1$ (L)	% Change
Baseline	2.05	
Diluent	1.98	
1.25 mg/ml	1.55	−22

ules; some begin at higher doses in order to shorten the length of a test. One recommended dosing schedule that reduces the number of doses and thus shortens the procedure time is that when the FEV$_1$ is greater than 80% of predicted and falls by less than 10% after the diluent inhalation, the starting concentration can be mg/ml in patients on no medication, 0.25 mg/ml in those on bronchodilators, and 0.125 in those on steroids. In all other instances the starting concentration should be 0.03 mg/ml.[9] Although these guidelines are assumed to be safe and help to shorten the duration of a bronchial challenge, they may not hold true for all patients. I recommend that laboratories performing methacholine or histamine challenges use dosing schedules from published articles and start at the lowest dose. If modified dosing schedules that shorten the procedure are desired, use caution and stay with published schedules.

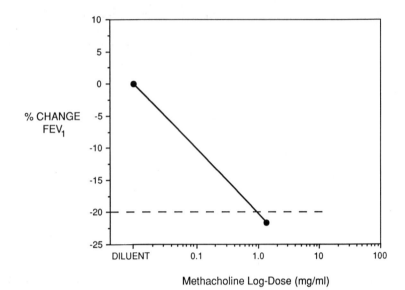

Figure 5.11. Graphic representation of methacholine challenge on the 10-year-old boy in Case 5.1.

Table 5.3: Pulmonary function tests (spirometry and specific conductance) showing the highest baseline and postdiluent FEV$_1$, and average baseline and postdiluent SGaw

	Baseline	Diluent
FVC (L)	3.89 (104)*	3.91
FEV$_1$ (L)	3.21 (102)	3.19
FEV$_1$/FVC (%)	83	82
SGaw	0.25	0.24

*Values in parentheses are percent predicted.

CASE 5.2

A 32-year-old avid woman runner was scheduled for a methacholine challenge because she noticed that she was wheezing and was more short of breath after some recent runs. She was not on any medications and had no history of pulmonary problems. After performing the baseline tests, the diluent saline was administered; the results are shown in Table 5.3.

Question:
What would be a reasonable starting methacholine dose?

**Table 5.4: Results of spirometry and specific conductance from metha-
choline challenge showing percent change from the postdiluent values**

	FEV1	%Change	SGaw	%Change
Baseline	3.21		0.25	
Diluent	3.19	−1**	0.24	−4
1.25 mg/ml	3.13	−2	0.18	−25
2.50	2.90	−9	0.15	−38
5.00	2.43	−24	0.11	−54

**Percent change is calculated from postdiluent values and the highest FEV1 within a series of efforts.

Answer and Discussion:

It would not be unreasonable to start at a very low dose such as <0.5 mg/ml. However, given her very normal PFTs and the fact that she does not take any pulmonary medications, a higher dose would be more reasonable and would shorten the duration of the test. One protocol that is commonly used is to start at a concentration of approximately 1.25 mg/ml in patients whose FEV_1 is above 80% predicted and falls by less than 10% after diluent inhalation, and the patient is on no pulmonary medications. If this patient were on bronchodilators, the starting dose would be much lower (e.g., 0.2 to 0.3 mg/ml).

The challenge was started and the results are shown in Table 5.4 and Figure 5.12.

Question:

What is the interpretation of the methacholine challenge?

Answer and Discussion:

The methacholine challenge is positive, as the FEV_1 fell by more than 20% and specific conductance (SGaw) fell by more than 40% after the 5 mg/ml dose. The $PC_{20}FEV_1$ was calculated as follows:

$$\log X = \log X_1 + \frac{(Y - Y_1)(X_2 - X_1)}{(Y_2 - Y_1)}$$

where,

$X \ = \ PC_{20}FEV_1$
$X_1 \ = \ $ log dose preceding the dose that caused a 20% fall
$X_2 \ = \ $ log dose that caused a 20% fall
$Y \ = \ $ 80% of postdiluent FEV_1
$Y_1 \ = \ FEV_1$ of dose preceding the dose that caused a 20% fall
$Y_2 \ = \ FEV_1$ of dose that caused a 20% fall

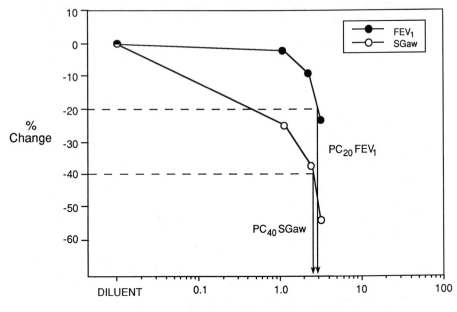

Figure 5.12. Graphic representation of methacholine challenge on the 32-year-old woman in Case 5.2 showing the provocative concentrations for FEV_1 and SGaw.

$$\log PC_{20}FEV_1 = \log 2.5 + \frac{(2.55 - 2.90)(\log 5.0 - \log 2.5)}{(2.43 - 2.90)}$$

$$\log PC_{20}FEV_1 = 0.398 + \frac{(-0.35)(0.699 - 0.398)}{(-0.47)}$$

$$\log PC_{20}FEV_1 = 0.398 + 0.224$$
$$\log PC_{20}FEV_1 = 0.622$$
$$PC_{20}FEV_1 = 4.19 \text{ mg/ml}$$

A $PC_{20}FEV_1$ of 4.19 mg/ml would be a mild sensitivity.

REFERENCES

1. Boushey HA, Holtzman MJ, Sheller JR, Nadel JA. State of the art: bronchial hyperreactivity. Am Rev Respir Dis 1980; 121:389–413.
2. Anderson SD. Exercise-induced asthma: the state of the art. Chest 1985;5(suppl): 191–195.
3. Bhagat RG, Grunstein MM. Comparison of responsiveness to methacholine, histamine, and exercise in subgroups of asthmatic children. Am Rev Respir Dis 1984;129:221–224.
4. Chatham M, Bleeker ER, Smith PL, et al. A comparison of histamine, methacho-

line, and exercise airway reactivity in normal and asthmatic subjects. Am Rev Respir Dis 1982;126:235–240.

5. Eggleston PA. A comparison of the asthmatic response to methacholine and exercise. J Allergy Clin Immunol 1979;63: 104–110.

6. Anderton RC, Cuff MT, Frith PA, et al. Bronchial responsiveness to inhaled histamine and exercise. J Allergy Clin Immunol 1979;63:315–320.

7. Kiviloog J. Bronchial reactivity to exercise and metachoine [sic] in bronchial asthma. Scand J Resp Dis 1973;54:347–358.

8. Mellis CM, Kattan M, Keens TG, Levison H. Comparative study of histamine and exercise challenges in asthmatic children. Am Rev Respir Dis 1978;117:911–915.

9. Hargreave FE, Ryan A, Thomson NC, et al. Bronchial responsiveness to histamine or methacholine in asthma: measurement and clinical significance. J Allergy Clin Immunol 1981;68:347–355.

10. Malo JL, Pineau L, Cartier A, Martin RR. Reference values of the provocative concentrations of methacholine that cause 6% and 20% changes in forced expiratory volume in one second in a normal population. Am Rev Respir Dis 1983;128:8–11.

11. Juniper EF, Frith PA, Dunnett C, et al. Reproducibility and comparison of responses to inhaled histamine and methacholine. Thorax 1978;33:705–710.

12. Spector SL, Farr RS. A comparison of methacholine and histamine and histamine inhalations in asthmatics. J Allergy Clin Immunol 1975;56:308–316.

13. MacDonald NC, Whitmore CK, Makoid MC, Cobby J. Stability of methacholine chloride in bronchial provocation test solutions. Am J Hosp Pharm 1981;38: 868–870.

14. Pratter MR, Woodman TF, Irwin RS, Johnson B. Stability of stored methacholine chloride solutions. Am Rev Respir Dis 1982;128:717–719.

15. Subcommittee on Bronchial Inhalation Challenges. Guidelines for bronchial inhalation challenges with pharmacologic and antigenic agents. ATS News 1980; Spring:11–19.

16. Chai H, Farr RS, Forehlich LA, et al. Standardization of bronchial inhalation challenge procedures. J Allergy Clin Immunol 1975;56:323–327.

17. Cockcroft DW, Killian DN, Melton JJA, et al. Bronchial reactivity to inhaled histamine: a method and clinical survey. Clin Allergy 1977;7:235–243.

18. Ryan G, Dolovich MB, Obminski G, et al. Standardization of inhalation provocation tests: influence of nebulizer output, particle size, and method of inhalation. J Allergy Clin Immunol 1981;67: 156–161.

19. Massey DG, Miyauchi D, Fournier-Massey G. Nebulizer function. Bull Eur Physiopathol Respir 1982;18:257–275.

20. Ryan G, Dolovich MB, Roberts RS, et al. Standardization of inhalation provocation tests, two techniques of aerosol generation and inhalation compared. Am Rev Respir Dis 1981;123:195–199.

21. Yan K, Salome C, Woolcock AJ. Rapid method for measurement of bronchial responsiveness. Thorax 1983;38:760–765.

22. Chatham M, Bleecker ER, Norman P, et al. A screening test for airways reactivity; an abbreviated methacholine inhalation challenge. Chest 1982;82:15–18.

23. Corrao WM, Braman SS, Irwin RS. Chronic cough as the sole presenting manifestation of bronchial asthma. N Eng J Med 1979;300:633–637.

24. European Society for Clinical Respiratory Physiology (SECPR) Working Group on Bronchial Hyperreactivity. Guidelines for standardization of bronchial challenges with (nonspecific) bronchoconstricting agents. Bull Europ Physiopath Resp 1983;19:495–514.

25. Spector S, Luparello TJ, Koepetzky MT, et al. Response of asthmatics to methacholine and suggestion. Am Rev Respir Dis 1976;113:43–50.

26. Horton DJ, Suda WL, Kinsman RA, et al. Bronchoconstrictive suggestion in asthma: a role for airways hyperreactivity and emotions. Am Rev Respir Dis 1978;117:1029–1038.

27. Luparello T, Lyons HA, Bleecker ER, McFadden ER. Influences of suggestion on airway reactivity in asthmatic subjects. Psychosomat Med 1968;30:819–825.

28. Cartier A, Malo JL, Begin P, et al. Time course of the bronchoconstriction in-duced by inhaled histamine and methacholine. J Appl Physiol 1983;54:821–826.

29. Hargreave FE, Dolovich J, Boulet LP. Inhalation provocation tests. Sem Resp Med 1983;4:224–235.

SELF-ASSESSMENT QUESTIONS

1. The following results are from a methacholine challenge.

Dose	FEV$_1$
Baseline	3.10
Diluent	3.02
0.07 mg/ml	2.93
0.15 mg/ml	2.81
0.31 mg/ml	2.79
0.62 mg/ml	2.48
1.25 mg/ml	2.30

These results are consistent with:
   a. incomplete challenge
   b. positive challenge at 1.25 mg/ml
   c. positive challenge at 0.62 mg/ml
   d. negative challenge

2. Which of the following is not an indication for performing a methacholine challenge?
   a. to diagnose asthma
   b. to document the severity of hyperresponsive airways
   c. to test response to bronchodilator
   d. to follow changes in hyperresponsive airways

3. Innervation of the airway smooth muscle is accomplished by:
   a. parasympathetic nerves
   b. sympathetic nerves
   c. spinal nerves
   d. adrenergic nerves

4. All of the following are technical factors affecting response to challenge aerosol inhalation except:
   a. starting lung volume at time of inhalation
   b. expiratory flow rate
   c. breathhold time
   d. inspiratory flow rate

5. The minimum change in FEV_1 that qualifies a challenge as positive is:
   a. 15%
   b. 35%
   c. 10%
   d. 20%

6. A patient's FEV_1 falls 14% from baseline after inhalation of the diluent (saline) prior to a methacholine challenge. You should:
   a. repeat the FEV_1 after a 10-minute rest
   b. repeat the inhalation of diluent
   c. cancel the test
   d. proceed to the first methacholine dose

7. The provocative concentration is calculated from
   a. linear interpolation of the log dose
   b. slope of the dose function
   c. slope of the percent change time
   d. the threshold point

8. All of the following about the French-Rosenthal dosimeter are true except:
   a. it consists of an electronic variable time circuit
   b. it consists of an electronic variable flow circuit
   c. the valve opening is activated by inspiration
   d. it allows air to flow to a nebulizer for a fixed period of time

9. The following results are from a methacholine challenge:

Dose	FEV_1
Baseline	4.55
Diluent	4.49
0.31 mg/ml	4.23
0.62 mg/ml	4.18
1.25 mg/ml	4.11
2.50 mg/ml	3.80
5.0 mg/ml	3.82
10.0 mg/ml	3.81
25.0 mg/ml	3.79

These results are consistent with:
   a. a positive methacholine challenge
   b. a normal response

    c. a mildly positive methacholine challenge
    d. an incomplete methacholine challenge

10. All of the following are criteria for postponing a bronchial challenge except:
    a. recent viral infection
    b. aerosolized bronchodilator used within past 2 hours
    c. methacholine challenge on previous day
    d. FEV_1 of 1.20 liters

11. Which of the following is recommended by the American Thoracic Society as the required pulmonary function parameter on bronchial challenge reports?
    a. FVC
    b. FEV_1
    c. SGaw
    d. PEFR
    e. all of above

12. When explaining the bronchial challenge test to a patient, one should:
    a. explain in detail to gain patient confidence and cooperation
    b. tell the patient that his/her breathing might get worse during the test
    c. tell the patient that his/her breathing might get better or worse or stay the same
    d. tell the patient he/she is going to inhale several types of bronchodilators to measure response.

Appendices

APPENDIX 1: Conversion of Volumes at ATPS to BTPS

$$V_{BTPS} = V_{ATPS} \times \frac{PB - PH_2O}{PB - 47} \times \frac{310}{273 + T}$$

where: V_{BTPS} = volume of gas at body temperature and pressure, saturated with water vapor

V_{ATPS} = volume of gas at ambient temperature and pressure, saturated with water vapor

PB = barometric pressure (mm Hg)

PH_2O = vapor pressure of water at ambient temperature T from Table 1

47 = vapor pressure of water (PH_2O) at 37°C

310 = absolute body temperature

T = ambient or room temperature

273 = absolute 0°C

Table 1: Vapor pressure of water (PH_2O)

°C	PH_2O (mm Hg)	°C	PH_2O (mm Hg)
10	9	21	19
11	10	22	20
12	11	23	21
13	11	24	22
14	12	25	24
15	13	26	25
16	14	27	27
17	15	28	28
18	15	29	30
19	16	30	32
20	18	31	34

Example calculation:

The forced vital capacity is 3.40 liters at ATPS (ambient temperature and pressure, saturated with water vapor) when room temperature is 23°C and PB is 700 mm Hg. The BTPS (body temperature and pressure, saturated with water vapor) equivalent is calculated in the following way:

$$V_{BTPS} = V_{ATPS} \frac{PB - PH_2O}{PB - 47} \times \frac{310}{273 + T}$$

$$V_{BTPS} = 3.40 \times \frac{700 - 21}{700 - 47} \times \frac{310}{273 - 23}$$

$$V_{BTPS} = 3.40 \times \frac{679}{653} \times \frac{310}{296}$$

$$V_{BTPS} = 3.40 \times 1.0398 \times 1.0473$$

$$V_{BTPS} = 3.40 \times 1.089$$

$$V_{BTPS} = 3.70 \text{ liters}$$

APPENDIX 2: Conversion of Volumes at ATPS to STPD:

$$V_{STPD} = V_{ATPS} \times \frac{PB - PH_2O}{760} \times \frac{273}{273 + T}$$

where: V_{STPD} = volume of gas at standard temperature and pressure, dry

V_{ATPS} = volume of gas at ambient temperature and pressure, saturated with water vapor

PB = barometric pressure

PH_2O = vapor pressure of water at T (see Appendix 1, Table 1)

273 = absolute 0°C

T = ambient or room temperature

Example calculation:

The volume in a collection bag is 11.5 liters at ATPS (ambient temperature and pressure, saturated with water vapor) when the room temperature is 24°C and the PB is 720 mm Hg. The STPD (standard temperature and pressure, dry) equivalent is calculated in the following way:

$$V_{STPD} = V_{ATPS} \frac{PB - PH_2O}{760} \times \frac{273}{273 + T}$$

$$V_{STPD} = 11.5 \times \frac{720 - 22}{760} \times \frac{273}{273 + 24}$$

$$V_{STPD} = 11.5 \times 0.918 \times 0.919$$

$$V_{STPD} = 11.5 \times 0.844$$

$$V_{STPD} = 9.71 \text{ liters}$$

APPENDIX 3: Conversion of Volumes at ATPD to STPD

$$V_{STPD} = V_{ATPD} \times \frac{PB}{760} \times \frac{273}{273 + T}$$

where: V_{STPD} = volume of gas at standard temperature and pressure, dry

V_{ATPD} = volume of gas at ambient temperature and pressure, dry

PB = barometric pressure (mm Hg)

273 = absolute 0°C

T = ambient or room temperature

760 = standard barometric pressure at sea level

Example calculation:

The inspired volume during a single breath diffusing capacity test is 2.85 liters at ATPD (ambient temperature and pressure, dry, since the inspired gas is stored in a cylinder) when the room temperature is 24°C and the barometric pressure (PB) is 705 mm Hg. The STPD (standard temperature and pressure, dry) equivalent is calculated the following way:

$$V_{STPD} = V_{ATPD} \times \frac{PB}{760} \times \frac{273}{273 + T}$$

$$V_{STPD} = 2.85 \times \frac{705}{760} \times \frac{273}{273 + 24}$$

$$V_{STPD} = 2.85 \times 0.928 \times 0.919$$

$$V_{STPD} = 2.85 \times 0.853$$

$$V_{STPD} = 2.43 \text{ liters}$$

APPENDIX 4: Adult Reference Populations, Methods, and Regression Equations for Spirometry and Lung Volumes

FVC

Reference Populations

Reference	Year	Race*	Age Range	No. Subjects	Sex	Method△	Location
Abramowitz	1965	B	20-54	51	M	WS	New Jersey
Coultas	1988	H	25-80	80	M	WS	New Mexico
Cherniack	1972	C	15-79	870	M	B	Canada
Crapo	1981	C	15-91	125	M	WS	Utah
Crapo	1990	H	25-75	116	M	RS	Utah, Calif.
DaCosta	1971	A	20-66	134	M	WS	Singapore
Jain	1969	I	15-40	188	M	NS	India
Knudson	1983	C	6-85	322	M	P	Arizona
Morris	1971	C	20-84	517	M	WS	Oregon
Mustafa	1977	B	15-74	623	M	B	Africa
Stinson	1981	B	20-92	219	M	P	Tennessee
Wanger	Unpub.	C	20-74	70	M	P	Colorado
Abramowitz	1965	B	15-54	20	F	WS	New Jersey
Coultas	1988	H	25-80	168	F	WS	New Mexico
Cherniack	1972	C	15-79	452	F	B	Canada
Crapo	1981	C	15-84	126	F	WS	Utah
Crapo	1990	H	20-80	143	F	RS	Utah, Calif.
DaCosta	1971	A	20-66	73	F	WS	Singapore
Knudson	1983	C	6-88	375	F	P	Arizona
Morris	1971	C	20-84	471	F	WS	Oregon
Stinson	1981	B	20-92	293	F	P	Tennessee
Wanger	Unpub.	C	20-80	139	F	P	Colorado

* A = Asian, B = Black, C = Caucasian, H = Hispanic, I = Indian
△ WS = Water-seal, B = Bellows, P = Pneumotach, RS = Rolling-seal, NS = Not stated

FVC (L): Regression equations for adults separated by race

Race	Reverence	Sex	Regression Equation	SEE
Asian	DaCosta, 1971	M	0.1038 (Hin) − 0.0105 (A) − 2.761	0.449
		F	0.0463 (Hin) − 0.0147 (A) + 0.006 (Wlbs) − 0.289	0.368
Black	Abramowitz, 1965	M	0.051 (Hcm) − 0.018 (A) − 3.82	0.46
		F	0.0457 (Hcm) − 0.007 (A) − 3.94	0.37
	Mustafa, 1977	M	0.0604 (Hcm) − 0.016 (A) − 6.14	NS
	Stinson, 1981	M	0.127 (Hin) − 0.02 (A) − 3.998	NS
		F	0.079 (Hin) − 0.018 (A) − 1.570	NS
Cauc.	Cherniack, 1972	M	0.121 (Hin) − 0.0136 (A) − 3.184	NS
		F	0.078 (Hin) − 0.015 (A) − 1.049	NS
	Crapo, 1981	M	0.06 (Hcm) − 0.0214 (A) − 4.65	0.644
		F	0.0491 (Hcm) − 0.0216 (A) − 3.59	0.39
	Knudson, 1983	M	0.0844 (Hcm) − 0.0298 (A) − 8.7818	NS
		F	0.0427 (Hcm) − 0.0174 (A) − 2.9001	NS
	Morris, 1971	M	0.148 (Hin) − 0.025 (A) − 4.241	0.74
		F	0.115 (Hin) − 0.024 (A) − 2.852	0.52
	Wanger, Unpub.	M	0.0872 (Hcm) − 0.0308 (A) − 8.8705	
		F	0.0563 (Hcm) − 0.0179 (A) − 4.6225	
Hisp.	Coultas, 1988	M	2.9247 (Hcm) − 6.6863	0.124
		F	2.8016 (Hcm) − 6.1478	0.124
	Crapo, 1990	M	0.0562 (Hcm) − 0.0313 (A) − 3.7883	0.524
		F	0.0413 (Hcm) − 0.0176 (A) − 2.5484	0.356

FEV$_1$
Reference Populations

Reference	Year	Race*	Age Range	No. Subjects	Sex	Method[Δ]	Location
Cherniack	1972	C	15-79	870	M	B	Canada
Coultas	1988	H	25-80	80	M	WS	New Mexico
Crapo	1981	C	15-91	125	M	WS	Utah
Crapo	1990	H	25-75	116	M	RS	Utah, Calif.
DaCosta	1971	A	20-66	134	M	WS	Singapore
Knudson	1983	C	6-85	322	M	P	Arizona

Morris	1971	C	20-84	517	M	WS	Oregon
Mustafa	1977	B	15-74	623	M	B	Africa
Stinson	1981	B	20-92	219	M	P	Tennessee
Wanger	Unpub.	C	20-75	70	M	P	Colorado
Coultas	1988	H	25-80	168	F	WS	New Mexico
Cherniack	1972	C	15-79	452	F	B	Canada
Crapo	1981	C	15-84	126	F	WS	Utah
Crapo	1990	H	20-80	143	F	RS	Utah, Calif.
DaCosta	1971	A	20-66	73	F	WS	Singapore
Knudson	1983	C	6-88	375	F	P	Arizona
Morris	1971	C	20-84	471	F	WS	Oregon
Stinson	1981	B	20-92	293	F	P	Tennessee
Wanger	Unpub.	C			F	P	Colorado

* A = Asian, B = Black, C = Caucasian, H = Hispanic, I = Indian
Δ WS = Water-seal, B = Bellows, P = Pneumotach, RS = Rolling-seal, NS = Not stated

FEV$_1$ (L):   Regression equations for adults separated by race

Race	Reference	Sex	Regression Equation	SEE
Asian	DaCosta, 1971	M	0.0678 (Hin) − 0.0189 (A) − 0.774	0.329
		F	0.0431 (Hin) − 0.0175 (A) + 0.232	0.278
Black	Mustafa, 1977	M	0.046 (Hcm) − 0.022 (A) − 3.864	0.41
	Stinson, 1981	M	0.096 (Hin) − 0.021 (A) − 3.998	NS
		F	0.063 (Hin) − 0.017 (A) − 0.951	NS
Cauc.	Cherniack, 1972	M	0.091 (Hin) − 0.0232 (A) − 1.507	NS
		F	0.060 (Hin) − 0.019 (A) − 0.187	NS
	Crapo, 1981	M	0.0414 (Hcm) − 0.0244 (A) − 2.190	0.486
		F	0.0342 (Hcm) − 0.0255 (A) − 1.578	0.326
	Knudson, 1983	M	0.0665 (Hcm) − 0.0292 (A) − 6.5147	NS
		F	0.0309 (Hcm) − 0.0201 (A) − 1.405	NS
	Morris, 1971	M	0.092 (Hin) − 0.032 (A) − 1.260	NS
		F	0.089 (Hin) − 0.025 (A) − 1.932	NS
	Wanger, Unpub.	M	0.0596 (Hcm) − 0.0223 (A) − 5.405	
		F	0.0425 (Hcm) − 0.0241 (A) − 2.880	
Hisp.	Coultas, 1988	M	3.77 (Hcm) − 0.029 (A) − 2.88	0.439

	F	3.21 (Hcm) $-$ 0.024 (A) $-$ 1.42	0.298
Crapo, 1990	M	0.0451 (Hcm) $-$ 0.0301 (A) $-$ 2.7721	0.446
	F	0.0378 (Hcm) $-$ 0.0361 (A) $-$ 0.0048 (Wkg) $-$ 2.14	0.296

FEF25-75%
Reference Populations

Reference	Year	Race*	Age Range	No. Subjects	Sex	Method△	Location
Cherniack	1972	C	15-79	870	M	B	Canada
Coultas	1988	H	25-80	80	M	WS	New Mexico
Crapo	1981	C	15-91	125	M	WS	Utah
Crapo	1990	H	25-75	116	M	RS	Utah, Calif.
Knudson	1983	C	6-85	322	M	P	Arizona
Morris	1971	C	20-84	517	M	WS	Oregon
Stinson	1981	B	20-92	219	M	P	Tennessee
Cherniack	1972	C	15-79	452	F	B	Canada
Coultas	1988	H	25-80	168	F	WS	New Mexico
Crapo	1981	C	15-84	126	F	WS	Utah
Crapo	1990	H	20-80	143	F	RS	Utah, Calif.
Knudson	1983	C	6-88	375	F	P	Arizona
Morris	1971	C	20-84	471	F	WS	Oregon
Stinson	1981	B	20-92	293	F	P	Tennessee

* A = Asian, B = Black, C = Caucasian, H = Hispanic, I = Indian
△ WS = Water-seal, B = Bellows, P = Pneumotach, RS = Rolling-seal, NS = Not stated

FEF25-75% (L/sec): Regression equations for adults separated by race

Race	Reference	Sex	Regression Equation	SEE
Black	Stinson, 1981	M	0.127 (Hin) $-$ 0.02 (A) $-$ 3.998	NS
		F	0.043 (Hin) $-$ 0.028 (A) $-$ 1.061	NS
Cauc.	Cherniack, 1972	M	0.059 (Hin) $-$ 0.037 (A) $+$ 2.611	NS
		F	0.049 (Hin) $-$ 0.031 (A) $+$ 2.256	NS
	Crapo, 1981	M	0.0204 (Hcm) $-$ 0.038 (A) $+$ 2.133	1.666
		F	0.0154 (Hcm) $-$ 0.046 (A) $+$ 2.683	0.792
	Knudson, 1983	M	0.0579 (Hcm) $-$ 0.0363 (A) $-$ 4.5175	NS

		F	0.0209 (Hcm) − 0.0344 (A) + 1.1277	NS
	Morris, 1971	M	0.047 (Hin) − 0.045 (A) + 2.513	NS
		F	0.060 (Hin) − 0.030 (A) + 0.551	NS
Hisp.	Coultas, 1988	M	2.072 (Hcm) − 0.044 (A) + 2.18	1.081
		F	1.96 (Hcm) − 0.036 (A) − 1.58	0.796
		M	0.0453 (Hcm) − 0.0389 (A) − 2.0574	1.130
		F	0.0330 (Hcm) − 0.0361 (A) − 0.3758	0.785

FEFmax, FEF25%, FEF50%, FEF75%
Reference Populations

Reference	Year	Race*	Age Range	No. Subjects	Sex	Method△	Location
Cherniack	1972	C	15-79	870	M	B	Canada
Knudson	1976	C	6-85	291	M	P	Arizona
Cherniack	1972	C	15-79	452	F	B	Canada
Knudson	1976	C	6-88	455	F	P	Arizona

* C = Caucasian,
△ B = Bellows, P = Pneumotach

FEFmax, FEF25%, FEF50%, FEF75%, (L/sec):   Adult Regression Equations

Race	Reference	Sex	Regression Equation	SEE
FEFmax				
Cauc.	Cherniack, 1972	M	0.144 (Hin) − 0.024 (A) + 0.225	NS
		F	0.091 (Hin) − 0.018 (A) + 1.132	NS
	Knudson, 1976	M	0.094 (Hcm) + 0.035 (A) − 5.993	
		F	0.049 (Hcm) − 0.025 (A) − 0.735	
FEF25%				
Cauc.	Cherniack, 1972	M	0.036 (Hin) − 0.041 (A) + 1.984	NS
		F	0.023 (Hin) − 0.034 (A) + 2.216	NS
	Knudson, 1976	M	0.088 (Hcm) − 0.035 (A) − 0.035	
		F	0.043 (Hcm) − 0.025 (A) − 0.132	
FEF50%				
Cauc.	Cherniack, 1972	M	0.065 (Hin) − 0.03 (A) + 2.403	NS
		F	0.062 (Hin) − 0.023 (A) + 1.426	NS
	Knudson, 1976	M	0.069 (Hcm) − 0.015 (A) − 5.40	
		F	0.035 (Hcm) − 0.013 (A) − 0.444	

FEF75%

Cauc.	Cherniack, 1972	M	0.090 (Hin) − 0.199 (A) + 2.726	NS
		F	0.069 (Hin) − 0.019 (A) + 2.147	NS
	Knudson, 1976	M	0.044 (Hcm) − 0.012 (A) − 4.143	
		F	− 0.014 (A) + 3.042	

FRC
Reference Populations

Reference	Year	Race*	Age Range	No. Subjects	Sex	Method$^\Delta$	Location
DaCosta	1971	A	20-66	134	M	Hel	Singapore
Goldman	1959	NS	NS	44	M	Hyd	S. Africa
Grimby	1963	NS	20-65	152	M	Hel	Sweden
Jain	1969	I	15-40	188	M		India
Wanger	Unpub.	C	20-75	70	M	BP	Colorado
Withers	1988	NS	18-79	162	M	Hel	Australia
DaCosta	1971	A	20-66	73	F	Hel	Singapore
Goldman	1959	NS		50	F	Hyd	S. Africa
Grimby	1963	NS	18-72	58	F	Hel	Sweden
Wanger	Unpub.	C	20-80	139	F	BP	Colorado

* A = Asian, C = Caucasian, I = Indian
$^\Delta$ Hyd = Hydrogen dilution, Hel = Helium dilution, BP = Body plethysmograph

FRC (L): Regression equations for adults separated by race

Race	Reference	Sex	Regression Equation	SEE
Asian	DaCosta, 1971	M	0.0608 (Hcm) − 0.0258 (Wkg) − 5.586	0.370
		F	0.0166 (Hcm) − 0.0174 (A) + 0.326	0.392
Cauc.	Wanger	M	0.0678 (Hcm) + 0.023 (A) − 9.156	
		F	0.0478 (Hcm) + 0.013 (A) − 5.444	
Indian	Jain	M	0.03664 (Hcm) + 0.008 (A) − 3.484	NS
NS	Goldman, 1959	M	0.081 (Hcm) − 1.792 (BSA) − 7.11	NS
		F	0.53 (Hcm) − 0.017 (Wkg) − 4.74	
	Grimby, 1963	M	5.30 (Hm) + 0.015 (A) − 0.037 (Wkg) − 3.89	NS

	F	5.13 (Hm) − 0.028 (Wkg) − 4.50	
Withers, 1988	M	0.0887 (Hcm) − 0.038 (Wkg) + 6.04	0.55
		(A) − 9.636	

TLC
Reference Population

Reference	Year	Race*	Age Range	No. Subjects	Sex	Method[Δ]	Location
DaCosta	1971	A	20-66	134	M	Hel	Singapore
Goldman	1959	NS	NS	44	M	Hyd	S. Africa
Grimby	1963	NS	20-65	152	M	Hel	Sweden
Jain	1969	I	15-40	188	M		India
Wanger	Unpub.	C	20-75	70	M	BP	Colorado
Withers	1988	NS	18-79	162	M	Hel	Australia
DaCosta	1971	A	20-66	73	F	Hel	Singapore
Goldman	1959	NS	NS	50	F	Hyd	S. Africa
Grimby	1963	NS	18-72	58	F	Hel	Sweden
Wanger	Unpub.	C	20-80	139	F	BP	Colorado

* A = Asian, C = Caucasian, I = Indian
[Δ] Hyd = Hydrogen dilution, Hel = Helium dilution, BP = Body plethysmograph

TLC (L): Regression equations for adults separated by race

Race	Reference	Sex	Regression Equation	SEE
Asian	DaCosta, 1971	M	0.1998 (Hin) − 7.934	
		F	0.0926 (Hin) − 0.0163 (A) − 1.203	
Cauc.	Wanger, Unpub.	M	0.1111 (Hcm) + 0.0130 (A) − 12.795	
		F	0.0779 (Hcm) − 0.0113 (A) − 7.662	
Indian	Jain, 1969	M	0.06679 (Hcm) + 0.0132 (A) − 5.075	
NS	Goldman, 1959	M	0.094 (Hcm) − 0.015 (A) − 9.167	
		F	0.079 (Hcm) − 0.008 (A) − 7.49	
	Grimby, 1963	M	6.92 (Hm) − 0.017 (Wkg) − 4.30	
		F	6.71 (Hm) − 0.015 (A) − 5.77	
	Withers, 1988	M	0.1029 (Hcm) − 0.01546 (Wkg) − 10.171	

RV
Reference Population

Reference	Year	Race*	Age Range	No. Subjects	Sex	Method△	Location
DaCosta	1971	A	20-66	134	M	Hel	Singapore
Goldman	1959	NS	NS	44	M	Hyd	S. Africa
Grimby	1963	NS	20-65	152	M	Hel	Sweden
Jain	1969	I	15-40	188	M		India
Wanger	Unpub.	C	20-75	70	M	BP	Colorado
Withers	1988	NS	18-79	162	M	Hel	Australia
DaCosta	1971	A	20-66	73	F	Hel	Singapore
Goldman	1959	NS	NS	50	F	Hyd	S. Africa
Grimby	1963	NS	18-72	58	F	Hel	Sweden
Wanger	Unpub.	C	20-80	139	F	BP	Colorado

* A = Asian, C = Caucasian, I = Indian
△ Hyd = Hydrogen dilution, Hel = Helium dilution, BP = Body plethysmograph

RV (L): Regression equations for adults separated by race

Race	Reference	Sex	Regression Equation	SEE
Asian	DaCosta, 1971	M	0.1137 (Hin) $+ 0.0116$ (A) $- 0.0076$ (Wlbs) $- 5.392$	
		F	0.0124 (Hin) $- 0.740$	
Cauc.	Wanger, Unpub.	M	0.019 (Hcm) $+ 0.0409$ (A) $- 2.952$	
		F	0.0235 (Hcm) $- 0.0257$ (A) $- 3.255$	
Indian	Jain, 1969	M	0.06679 (Hcm) $+ 0.0132$ (A) $- 5.075$	
NS	Goldman, 1959	M	0.027 (Hcm) $- 0.017$ (A) $- 3.447$	
		F	0.032 (Hcm) $- 0.009$ (A) $- 3.90$	
	Grimby, 1963	M	1.98 (Hm) $- 0.015$ (Wkg) $+ 0.022$ (A) $- 1.54$	
		F	2.68 (Hm) $+ 0.007$ (A) $- 3.42$	
	Withers, 1988	M	0.0349 (Hcm) $+ 0.0189$ (A) $- 0.0097$ (Wkg) $- 4.64$	

REFERENCES

Abramowitz S, Leiner GC, Lewis WA, Small MJ. Vital capacity in the negro. Am Rev Respir Dis 1965;92;287–292.

Cherniack RM, Raber MB. Normal standards for ventilatory function using an automated wedge spirometer. Am Rev Respir

Dis 1972;106:38–46.

Coultas DB, Howard CA, Skipper BJ, Samet JM. Spirometric prediction equations for hispanic children and adults in New Mexico. Am Rev Respir Dis 1988;138:1386–1392.

Crapo RO, Jensen RL, Lockey JE, Aldrich V, Elliott CG. Normal spirometric values in healthy Hispanic Americans. Chest 1990; 98:1435–1439.

Crapo RO, Morris AH, Gardner RM. Reference spirometric values using techniques and equipment that meet ATS recommendations. Am Rev Respir Dis 1981;123:659–664.

DaCosta JL. Pulmonary function studies in healthy Chinese adults in Singapore. Am Rev Respir Dis 1971;104:128–131.

Goldman HL, Becklake MR. Respiratory function tests. Am Rev Tuberc 1959;79:457–467.

Grimby G, Soderholm B. Spirometric studies in normal subjects. Acta Medica Scand 1963;173:199–206.

Jain SK, Ramiah TJ. Normal standards of pulmonary function tests for healthy Indian men 15–40 years old: comparison of different regression equations (predicted formulae). Ind Jour Med Res 1969;57:1453–1466.

Knudson RJ, Lebowitz MD, Holberg CJ, Burrows B. Changes in the normal expiratory flow-volume curve with growth and aging. Am Rev Respir Dis 1983;127:725–734.

Knudson RJ, Slatin RC, Lebowitz MD, Burrows B. The maximal expiratory flow-volume curve. Am Rev Respir Dis 1976;113:587–600.

Morris JF, Koski A, Johnson LC. Spirometric standards for healthy nonsmoking adults. Am Rev Respir Dis 1971;103:57–67.

Mustafa KY. Spirometric lung function tests in normal men of African ethnic origin. Am Rev Respir Dis 1977;116:209–213.

Stinson JM, McPherson GL, Hicks K, et al. Spirometric standards for healthy black adults. J Nat Med Ass 1981;73:729–733.

Withers RT, Bourdon PC, Crockett A. Lung volume standards for healthy male lifetime nonsmokers. Chest 1988;92:91–97.

APPENDIX 5: Mathematics of Boyle's Law

$$P_1V_1 = P_2V_2$$

if, $P_2 = P + \Delta P$ and $V_2 = V + \Delta V$, then

$$PV = (P + \Delta P)(V + \Delta V)$$

where,   P   = alveolar pressure
ΔP = change in pressure during panting against shutter
V   = thoracic gas volume (usually at FRC)
ΔV = change in FRC due to compression and decompression

$$PV = PV + P\Delta V + \Delta PV + \Delta P\Delta V$$

where, $\Delta P\Delta V$ can be omitted because it is relatively small, then

$$PV = PV + P\Delta V + \Delta PV$$

$$0 = P\Delta V + \Delta PV$$

$$\Delta PV = -P\Delta V$$

$$V = \frac{-P\Delta V}{\Delta P} \text{ where the negative sign is ignored}$$

where, P = alveolar pressure
  ΔV = change in body box volume when panting
  ΔP = change in alveolar pressure (measured at mouth) when
    panting against closed shutter
  V = thoracic gas volume when shutter is closed, usually FRC

APPENDIX 6: Lung Function Regression Equations for Children

FVC

1. Polger, Promadhat, 1971:

  Males: FVC (L) = $4.4 \times 10^{-6} \times$ (Htcm)$^{2.67}$
  Females: FVC (L) = $3.3 \times 10^{-6} \times$ (Htcm)$^{2.72}$

2. Dickman, Schmidt, Gardner: 1971, age range 5–18, 482 males and 468 females:

  Males, 42–59 inches: FVC (L) = 0.094 (Hin) − 3.042
    60–78 inches: FVC (L) = 0.174 (A) + 0.164 (Hin) − 9.425

  Females, 42–59 inches: FVC (L) = 0.077 (Hin) − 2.371
    60–78 inches: FVC (L) = 0.102 (A) + 0.117 (Hin) − 5.869

3. Hsu, Jenkins, Hsi, et al.: 1979, age range 7–19, 558 Hispanics, 720 whites, and 527 blacks:

  Males, Hispanic: FVC (ml) = $1.06 \times 10^{-3} \times$ (Htcm)$^{2.97}$
    black: FVC (ml) = $1.07 \times 10^{-3} \times$ (Htcm)$^{2.83}$
    white: FVC (ml) = $3.58 \times 10^{-4} \times$ (Htcm)$^{3.18}$

  Females, Hispanic: FVC (ml) = $1.25 \times 10^{-3} \times$ (Htcm)$^{2.92}$
    black: FVC (ml) = $8.34 \times 10^{-4} \times$ (Htcm)$^{2.98}$
    white: FVC (ml) = $2.57 \times 10^{-3} \times$ (Htcm)$^{2.78}$

FEV$_1$

1. Polger, Promadhat, 1971:

  Males: FEV$_1$ (ml) = $2.1 \times 10^{-5} \times$ (Htcm)$^{2.8}$
  Females: FEV$_1$ (ml) = $2.1 \times 10^{-5} \times$ (Htcm)$^{2.8}$

2. Dickman, Schmidt, Gardner: 1971, age range 5–18, 482 males and 468 females:

  Males, 42–59 inches: FEV$_1$ (L) = 0.085 (Htin) − 2.855

60–78 inches: FEV_1 (L) = 0.121 (A) + 0.143 (Htin) − 7.864

Females, 42–59 inches: FEV_1 (L) = 0.074 (Htin) − 2.482
60–78 inches: FEV_1 (L) = 0.085 (A) + 0.10 (Htin) − 4.939

3. Hsu, Jenkins, Hsi, et al.: 1979, age range 7–19, 558 Hispanics, 720 whites, and 527 blacks:

Males, Hispanic: FEV_1 (ml) = 1.73 × 10^{-3} × $(Htcm)^{2.85}$
black: FEV_1 (ml) = 1.03 × 10^{-3} × $(Htcm)^{2.92}$
white: FEV_1 (ml) = 7.74 × 10^{-4} × $(Htcm)^{3.00}$

Females, Hispanic: FEV_1 (ml) = 1.61 × 10^{-3} × $(Htcm)^{2.85}$
black: FEV_1 (ml) = 1.14 × 10^{-3} × $(Htcm)^{2.89}$
white: FEV_1 (ml) = 3.79 × 10^{-3} × $(Htcm)^{2.68}$

FEF25–75

1. Polger, Promadhat, 1971:

Males: FEF25–75 (L/S) = [− 207.7 + 2.621 (Htcm)] / 60
Females: FEF25–75 (L/S) = [− 207.7 + 2.621 (Htcm)] / 60

2. Dickman, Schmidt, Gardner: 1971, age range 5–18, 482 males and 468 females:

Males, 42–59 inches: FEF25–75 (L/S) = 0.094 (Htin) − 2.614
60–78 inches: FEF25–75 (L/S) = 0.126 (A) + 0.135 (Htin) − 6.498

Females, 42–59 inches: FEF25–75 (L/S) = 0.087 (Htin) − 2.389
60–78 inches: FEF25–75 (L/S) = 0.083 (A) + 0.093 (Htin) − 3.499

3. Hsu, Jenkins, Hsi, et al.: 1979, age range 7–19, 558 Hispanics, 720 whites, and 527 blacks:

Males, Hispanic: FEF25–75 (ml/S) = 9.13 × 10^{-4} × $(Htcm)^{2.45}$
black: FEF25–75 (ml/S) = 3.61 × 10^{-4} × $(Htcm)^{2.60}$
white: FEF25–75 (ml/S) = 7.98 × 10^{-4} × $(Htcm)^{2.46}$

Females, Hispanic: FEF25–75 (ml/S) = 1.20 × 10^{-3} × $(Htcm)^{2.46}$
black: FEF25–75 (ml/S) = 1.45 × 10^{-3} × $(Htcm)^{2.34}$
white: FEF25–75 (ml/S) = 3.79 × 10^{-3} × $(Htcm)^{2.48}$

PEFR

1. Polger, Promadhat, 1971:

Males: PEFR (L/M) = − 425.57 + 5.2428 (Htcm)
Females: PEFR (L/M) = − 425.57 + 5.2428 (Htcm)

2. Hsu, Jenkins, Hsi, et al.: 1979, age range 7–19, 558 Hispanics, 720 whites, and 527 blacks:

Males, Hispanic: $PEFR\ (L/M) = 7.69 \times 10^{-4} \times (Htcm)^{2.63}$
  black: $PEFR\ (L/M) = 1.74 \times 10^{-4} \times (Htcm)^{2.92}$
  white: $PEFR\ (L/M) = 3.35 \times 10^{-4} \times (Htcm)^{2.78}$

Females, Hispanic: $PEFR\ (L/M) = 6.97 \times 10^{-4} \times (Htcm)^{2.64}$
  black: $PEFR\ (L/M) = 5.51 \times 10^{-4} \times (Htcm)^{2.68}$
  white: $PEFR\ (L/M) = 2.58 \times 10^{-3} \times (Htcm)^{2.37}$

FRC

1. Polger, Promadhat, 1971:

Males: $FRC\ (ml) = 0.75 \times 10^{-3} \times (Htcm)^{2.92}$
Females: $FRC\ (ml) = 1.78 \times 10^{-3} \times (Htcm)^{2.74}$

TLC

1. Polger, Promadhat, 1971:

Males: $TLC\ (ml) = 5.6 \times 10^{-3} \times (Htcm)^{2.67}$
Females: $TLC\ (ml) = 4.0 \times 10^{-3} \times (Htcm)^{2.73}$

REFERENCES

1. Polger G, Promadhat V. Pulmonary function testing in children: techniques and standards. Philadelphia: WB Saunders, 1971.
2. Dickman ML, Schmidt CD, Gardner RM. Spirometric standards for normal children and adolescents. Am Rev Respir Dis 1971;104:680–687.
3. Hsu KHK, Jenkins DE, Hsi BP, et al. Ventilatory functions of normal children and young adults—Mexican-American, White, and Black. Pediatrics 1979;95;14–23.

APPENDIX 7: Reference Equations for Exercise Testing

OXYGEN CONSUMPTION (L/M) AT MAXIMUM EXERCISE

1. Jones, Makrides, Hitchcock, et al., 1985, Ergometer

Males: $VO_2\ (L/M) = 0.034\ (Htcm) - 0.028\ (A) + 0.022\ (Wkg) - 3.76$
Females: $VO_2\ (L/M) = 0.025\ (Htcm) - 0.018\ (A) + 0.010\ (Wkg) - 2.26$

2. Wasserman, Hansen, Sue, Whipp, 1986, Ergometer

Males: $VO_2\ (ml/M) = Wkg\ [50.72 - 0.372\ (A)]$, not overweight
  $VO_2\ (ml/M) = [0.79\ (Htcm) - 60.7] \times [50.72 - 0.372\ (A)]$,
  overweight — $W > [0.79\ (Htcm) - 60.7]$

Females: VO_2 (ml/M) = $(42.8 + Wkg) \times [22.78 - 0.17 (A)]$, not overweight
VO_2 (ml/M) = $Htcm \times [14.81 - 0.11 (A)]$, overweight — W > $[0.65 (Htcm) - 42.8]$

3. Wasserman, Hansen, Sue, Whipp, 1986, Treadmill

Males: VO_2 (ml/M) = $Wkg [56.36 - 0.413 (A)]$, not overweight
VO_2 (ml/M) = $[0.79 (Htcm) - 60.7] \times [56.36 - 0.413 (A)]$, overweight — W > $[0.79 (Hcm) - 60.7]$

Females: VO_2 (ml/M) = $Wkg \times [44.37 - 0.413 (A)]$, not overweight
VO_2 (ml/M) = $[0.79 (Htcm) - 68.2] \times [44.37 - 0.413 (A)]$, overweight — W > $[0.79 (Htcm) - 68.2]$

MAXIMAL POWER OUTPUT (Kpm/min)*

1. Jones, Makrides, Hitchcock, et al., 1985, Ergometer

Males: Power Output = $25.3 (Htcm) - 9.06 (A) - 2759$
Females: Power Output = $9.5 (Htcm) - 9.21 (A) + 6.1 (Wkg) - 2759$

* Note—Kilopondmeter per minute (Kpm/min) = 9.8/60 watts, or 6 Kpm/min is about 1 watt.

MAXIMAL HEART RATE (beats/min)

1. Jones, Makrides, Hitchcock, et al., 1985, Ergometer

Males: Heart rate = $206 - 0.8 (A)$
Females: Heart rate = $198 - 0.63 (A)$

OXYGEN PULSE AT MAXIMUM EXERCISE (ml/beat)

1. Jones, Makrides, Hitchcock, et al., 1985, Ergometer

Males: Heart rate = $0.342 (Htcm) - 44.0$
Females: Heart rate = $0.190 (Htcm) - 21.4$

REFERENCES

1. Jones NL, Makrides L, Hitchcock C, et al. Normal standards for an incremental progressive cycle ergometer test. Am Rev Respir Dis 1985;131:700–708.

2. Wasserman K, Hansen JE, Sue DY, Whipp BJ. Principles of exercise testing and interpretation. Philadelphia: Lea & Febiger, 1986.

APPENDIX 8: How to Put Together a Procedure Manual for the Pulmonary Function Laboratory

A policy and procedure manual should be available for the pulmonary function laboratory. It should contain information about each test performed, personnel orientation, safety procedures, quality control, quality assurance, and other information as required by the accreditation agencies. The manual should be updated when procedures or equipment are modified or replaced and should be reviewed annually.

The sections of the manual that describe the testing procedures should be written by knowledgeable laboratory staff in language that would allow someone with much less knowledge to understand how to perform the tests. The format and organization I prefer and recommend follows below:

1. **Title Page:** The title page shows the department name, procedure name, date prepared and space for review "check-offs," and the signatures of the supervisor or manager and medical director. An example of a title page format that I use is shown in Figure A8.1.

2. **Principle.** This section contains a description of the purpose and the physiologic basis of the test. I sometimes include historical perspectives and other information (e.g., references and suggested reading) that I think will be valuable to the reader.

3. **Patient Preparation:** This section should contain a description of how the patient should be readied for the test including the withholding of medications or meals, smoking requirements (e.g., no smoking for 3 hours before test), clothing recommendations (e.g., shoes for walking), and contraindications for performing the test.

4. **Equipment and Supplies:** A list of all equipment and supplies that will be needed to perform the test, calculate the results, report the information, and clean up after the test is over. As an example, for spirometry this list might include:

   A. Brand X spirometer with pneumotach, computer, monitor, keyboard, and printer
   B. Breathing tube with cardboard mouthpiece
   C. Noseclip
   D. Computer paper
   E. Cold sterilization solution and large container
   E. Room thermometer and barometer
   F. Scale for height and weight
   G. Kleenex and wastebasket

5. **Equipment Set-Up and Calibration:** How to prepare the testing equipment for a test (e.g., check water level in spirometer, turn power on with I/O switch on front of instrument, or connect tubing to pneumotach), and how

calibration should be carried out and documented, including guidelines on limits of acceptability and frequency. As an example, for spirometry the description might read:

A. Turn main power switch on (located on front panel of computer).

B. Enter correct date, time, barometric pressure, and room temperature (°C)

C. Calibrate the pneumotach by selecting option 3 ("Calibrate") from Main Menu. Follow instructions prompted by computer for calibration.

D. Use 3-liter calibration syringe and withdraw/inject three times.

E. Vary the speed at which the 3-liter syringe plunger is moved when injecting and withdrawing volume.

F. Repeat calibration sequence and necessary adjustment until the calibration is accurate (i.e., values should be within ± 3% of the 3-liter syringe or 2.91 − 3.09 liters).

G. Print acceptable calibration results and store printout in calibration notebook.

6. **Procedure:** This section should have step-by-step directions on how to perform, measure, calculate, report the test results, and clean up. Frequently the instrument's operator manual contains much of this information.

7. **Reference Equations:** The current reference value equations and their journal references should be available. I also include other pertinent information with each equation such as age range reported, number of subjects, population criteria (e.g., race, locale).

8. **References:** A listing of any references used in preparation of the manual.

Figure A8.1: Example of title page for a testing procedure in Policy and Procedure Manual.

Department Procedure A
Page 1 of 10

DEPARTMENT: Pulmonary Function Laboratory
SUBJECT: Spirometry

PREPARED: February, 1990
REVIEWED: Date: _____   By: _____

_____   _____

_____   _____

_____   _____

_____   _____

_____

Manager

Medical Director

APPENDIX 9: Answers to self-assessment questions

Chapter 1

1. a	6. b
2. c	7. b
3. c	8. e
4. b	9. c
5. e	10. c

Chapter 2

1. c	6. b
2. b	7. a
3. b	8. d
4. c	9. e
5. a	10. c

Chapter 3

1. a	5. b
2. d	6. d
3. b	7. d
4. a	

Chapter 4

1. d	6. e	11. a
2. a	7. b	12. a
3. b	8. c	
4. a	9. a	
5. a	10. c	

Chapter 5

1. b	6. b	11. b
2. c	7. a	12. c
3. a	8. b	
4. b	9. b	
5. d	10. c	

Index

Page numbers in *italics* denote figures; those followed by "t" denote tables.